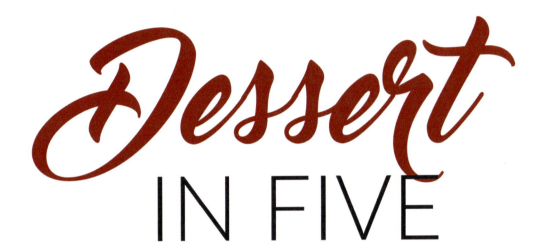

30 *low-carb* desserts

Up to **5** net carbs, **5** ingredients & **5** easy steps for every recipe

Vicky Ushakova and Rami Abramov

Table of Contents

About This Book 5

Keto 101 7
What Is Keto? 8
Calories & Macronutrients 10
A Nutritional Revolution 12
The Basics: Benefits of Going Keto 14
Steering Clear of the Keto Flu 16

Starting Keto 19
Part 1 — Out with the Old 20
Part 2 — In with the New! 22

Recipes 25
Notes 26
Raspberry Danish Cookies 28
Sugar-Free Nutella 30
Coconut Cream Pie 32
Cheesecake for One 34
Chocolate Peanut Butter Cups 36
Crazy for Coconut Cake 38
Macadamia Nut Clusters 40
Classic Crème Brûlée 42
Double Chocolate Mousse 44
Lemon Dream Bars 46
Avocado Chocolate Mousse 48
Stracciatella Gelato 50
Almond Fudge Brownies 52
Strawberries & Cream Pancakes 54
Cinnamon Mug Cake 56
Cookie Dough Mousse 58
Creamy Coconut Fudge 60
Banana Pudding 62
Sea Salt Chocolate Truffles 64
Double Lemon Jell-O Cake 66
Matcha Soufflé 68
Key Lime Panna Cotta 70
Maple Pecan Cookies 72
0-Carb Gummy Candy 74
Chocolate Haystack Cookies 76
White Chocolate Cashew Clusters 78
Strawberry Shortcake 80
Pumpkin Pudding 82
Mint Chocolate Chip Ice Cream 84
Banana Almond Muffins 86

Thank You 88
About the Authors 89
Personal Notes 91
References 98

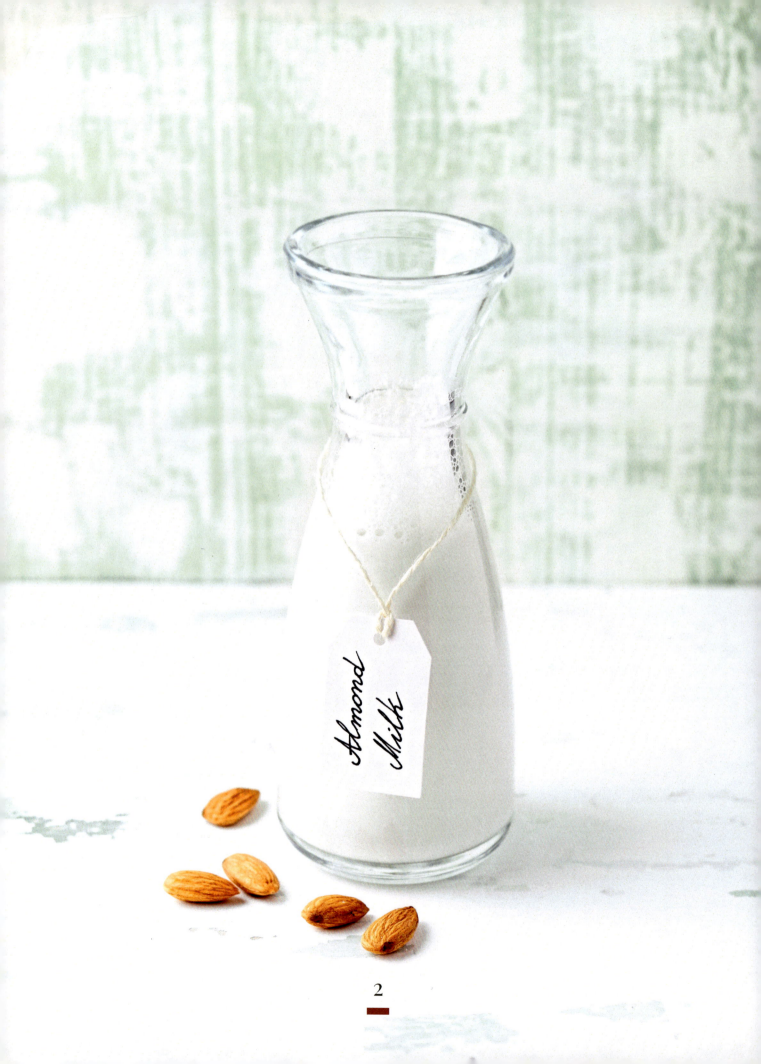

Disclaimer

Limit of Liability/Disclaimer of Warranty: Tasteaholics, Inc. is not a medical company or organization. Our books provide information in respect to healthy eating, nutrition and recipes and are intended for informational purposes only. We are not nutritionists or doctors and the information in this book and our website is not meant to be given as medical advice. We are two people sharing our success strategies and resources and encouraging you to do further research to see if they'll work for you too. Before starting any diet, you should always consult with your physician to rule out any health issues that could arise. Safety first, results second. Do not disregard professional medical advice or delay in seeking it because of this book.

Photography: © Kati Finell/Bigstock.com, p. 4; lisovskaya/Bigstock.com, p. 5; jirkaejc/Bigstock.com, p. 6; egal/Bigstock.com, p. 12; Madlen/Bigstock.com, p. 15; BelayaKaterina/Envato.com, p. 18; Nika111/Bigstock.com, p. 21; scukrov/Depositphotos.com, p. 21; zmaris/Depositphotos.com, p. 21; kornienkoalex/Depositphotos.com, p. 21; tashka2000/Bigstock.com, p. 22; ersler/Bigstock.com, p. 23; ivankmit/Envato.com, p. 24; janstarstud/Bigstock.com, p. 26; Valentina R./Bigstock.com, p. 30; Alex_star/elements.envato.com, p. 32; Yastremska/Bigstock.com, p. 34; seregam/elements.envato.com, p. 36; grafvision/elements.envato.com, p. 38; Inga Nielsen/Bigstock.com, p. 42; oysy/Bigstock.com, p. 44; sommai/Bigstock.com, p. 46; Kovaleva Katerina/Bigstock.com, p. 48; PeterHermesFurian/elements.envato.com, p. 52; magone/elements.envato.com, p. 54; Natika/Bigstock.com, p. 56; maxsol7/elements.envato.com, p. 58; Coprid/Bigstock.com, p. 60; 5_second/Bigstock.com, p. 62; picturepartners/elements.envato.com, p. 64; Denira777/Bigstock.com, p. 70; abracadabra99/Bigstock.com, p. 72; gresei/elements.envato.com, p. 78; Digidesign/Bigstock.com, p. 82; YVdavyd/elements.envato.com, p. 86; peetimus/Bigstock.com, p. 88; lenka/Bigstock.com, p. 88; barbaradudzinska/Bigstock.com, p. 89.

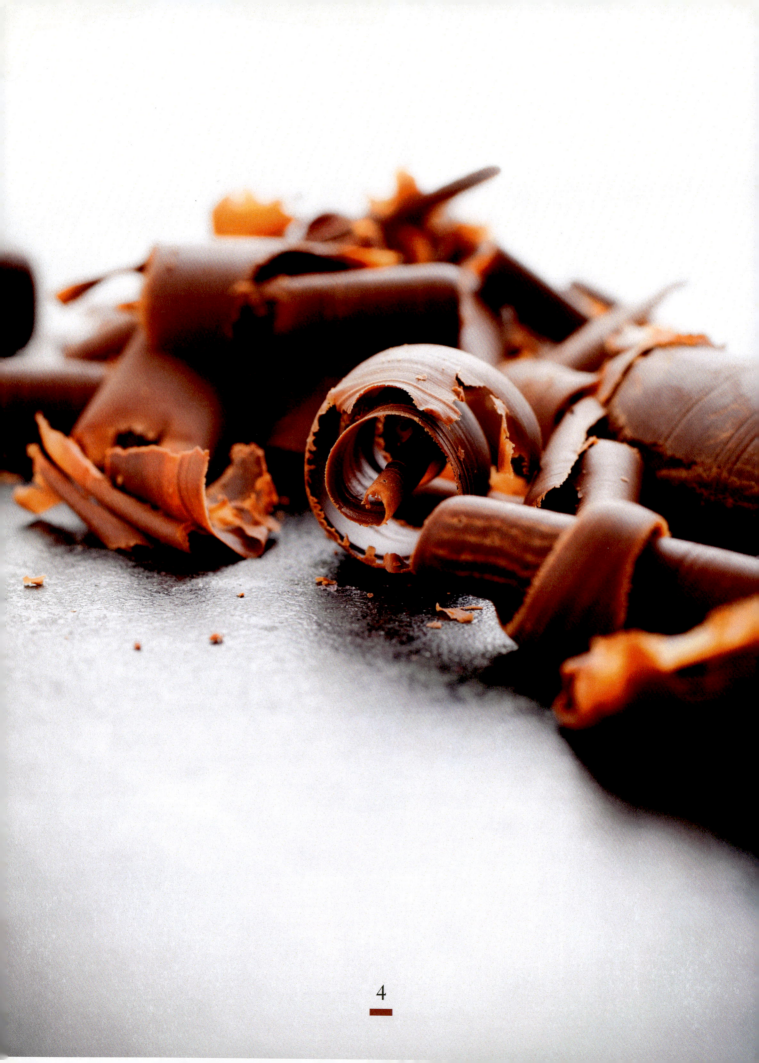

About This Book

This book was designed as a guide to help you kick start your ketogenic diet so you can lose weight, become healthy and have high energy levels every day.

Inside this book, you'll find the basics of the ketogenic diet, useful tips and delicious dessert recipes.

Each recipe is only 5 grams of net carbs or fewer and can be made with just 5 ingredients! There's nothing better than that.

Enjoy chocolate soufflés, strawberry cheesecakes, brownies, coconut cream pies, raspberry Danish cookies and much more every day of the month. Living a low-carb lifestyle has never been more enjoyable and sustainable!

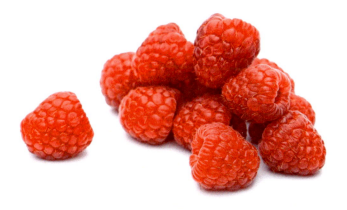

Let's get started!

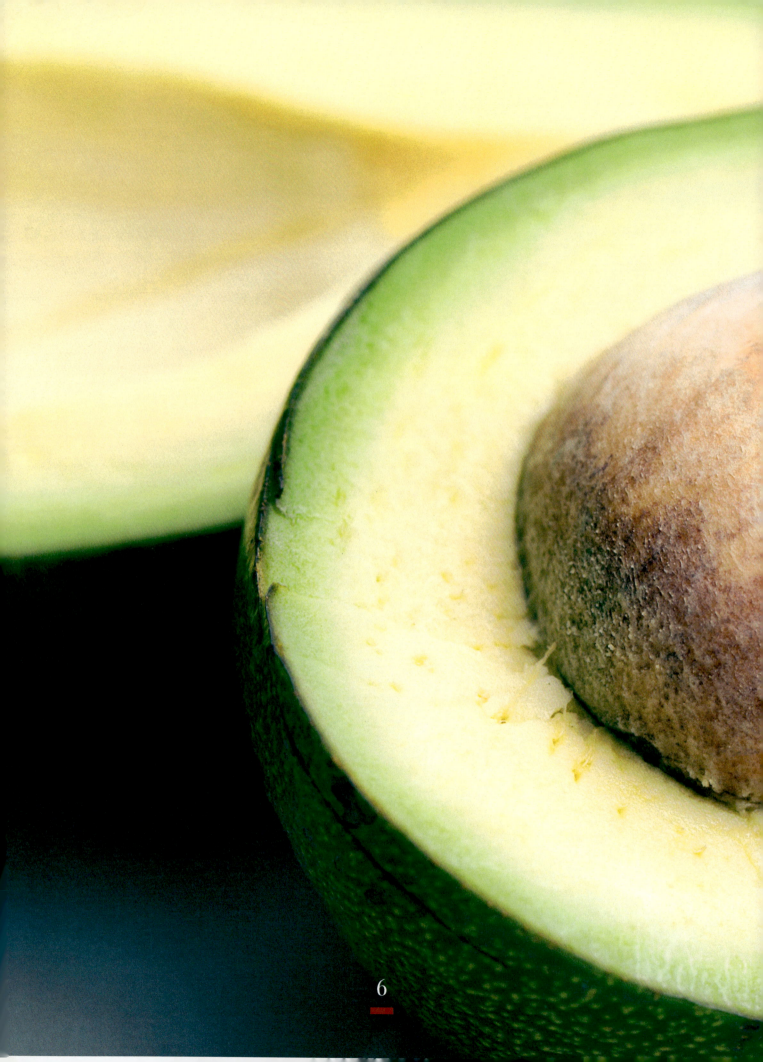

Keto 101

What Is Keto?

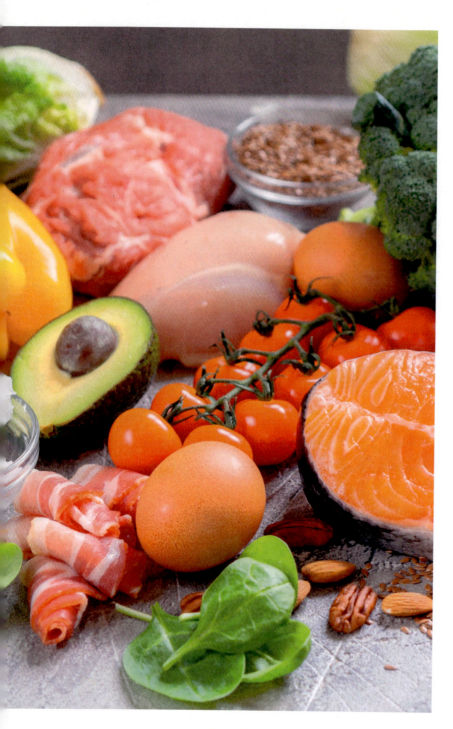

The Ketogenic Diet

The ketogenic (or keto) diet is a low-carbohydrate, high-fat diet. Maintaining this diet is a great tool for weight loss. More importantly, according to an increasing number of studies, it reduces risk factors for diabetes, heart diseases, stroke, Alzheimer's, epilepsy, and more.[1-6]

On the keto diet, your body enters a metabolic state called ketosis. While in ketosis your body is using ketone bodies for energy instead of glucose. Ketone bodies are derived from fat and are a much more stable, steady source of energy than glucose, which is derived from carbohydrates.

Entering ketosis usually takes anywhere from 3 days to a week. Once you're in ketosis, you'll be using fat for energy, instead of carbs. This includes the fat you eat and stored body fat.

While eating low-carb, you'll lose weight easier, feel satiated longer and enjoy consistent energy levels throughout your day.

Testing for Ketosis

You can test yourself to see whether you've entered ketosis just a few days after you've begun the keto diet! Use a *ketone urine test strip* and it will tell you the level of ketone bodies in your urine. If the concentration is high enough and the test strip shows any hue of purple, you've successfully entered ketosis!

The strips take only a few seconds to show results and are the fastest and most affordable way to check whether you're in ketosis.

Visit tasteaholics.com/strips and get a bottle of 100 test strips.

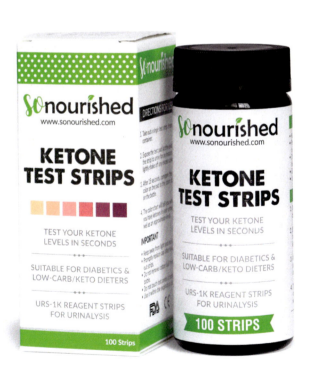

The Truth About Fat

You may be thinking, "but eating a lot of fat is bad!" The truth is, dozens of studies and meta studies with over 900,000 subjects have arrived at similar conclusions: eating saturated and monounsaturated fats have no effects on heart disease risks.[7,8]

Most fats are good and are essential to our health. Fats (fatty acids) and protein (amino acids) are essential for survival.

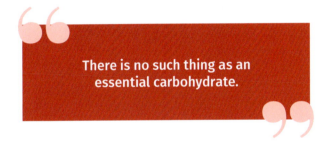

> There is no such thing as an essential carbohydrate.

Fats are the most efficient form of energy and each gram contains more than double the energy in a gram of protein or carbohydrates (more on that later).

The keto diet promotes eating fresh, whole foods like meat, fish, veggies, and healthy fats and oils as well as greatly reducing processed and chemically treated foods the Standard American Diet (SAD) has so long encouraged.

It's a diet that you can sustain long-term and enjoy. What's not to enjoy about bacon and eggs in the morning?

Calories & Macro-nutrients

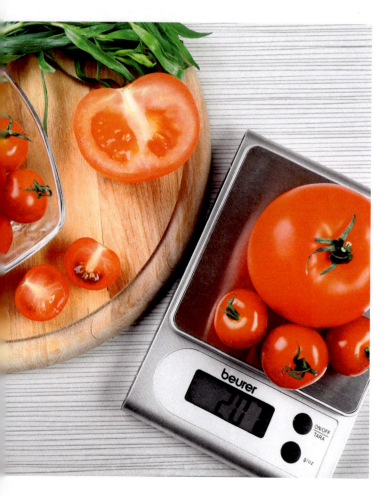

How Calories Work

A calorie is a unit of energy. When something contains 100 calories, it describes how much energy your body could get from consuming it. Calorie consumption dictates weight gain/loss.

If you burn an average of 1,800 calories and eat 2,000 calories per day, you will gain weight.

If you do light exercise that burns an extra 300 calories per day, you'll burn 2,100 calories per day, putting you at a deficit of 100 calories. Simply by eating at a deficit, you will lose weight because your body will tap into stored resources for the remaining energy it needs.

That being said, it's important to get the right balance of macronutrients every day so your body has the energy it needs.

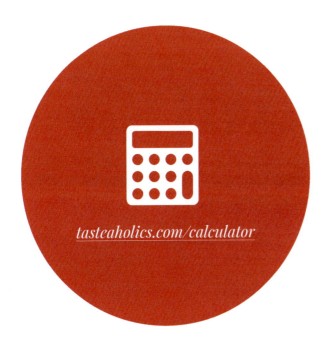

tasteaholics.com/calculator

What Are Macronutrients?

Macronutrients (macros) are molecules that our bodies use to create energy for themselves – primarily fat, protein and carbs. They are found in all food and are measured in grams (g) on nutrition labels.

- **Fat** provides 9 calories per gram
- **Protein** provides 4 calories per gram
- **Carbs** provide 4 calories per gram

Learn more at tasteaholics.com/macros.

Net Carbs

Most low-carb recipes write net carbs when displaying their macros. Net carbs are total carbs minus dietary fiber and sugar alcohols. Our bodies can't break them down into glucose so they don't count toward your total carb count.

Note: *Dietary fiber can be listed as soluble or insoluble.*

How Much Should You Eat?

On a keto diet, about 65 to 75 percent of the calories you consume daily should come from fat. About 20 to 30 percent should come from protein. The remaining 5 percent or so should come from carbohydrates.

Use our keto calculator to figure out exactly how many calories and macros you should be eating every day!

It will ask for basic information including your weight, activity levels and goals and instantly provide you with the total calories and grams of fat, protein and carbs that you should be eating each day.

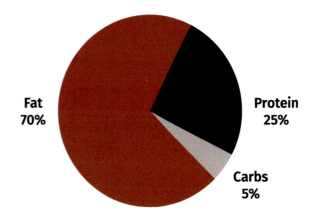

Note: *The calculator should be used as a general guideline. The results are based on your inputs and variables such as body fat percentage and basal metabolic rate are difficult to estimate correctly.*

A Nutritional Revolution

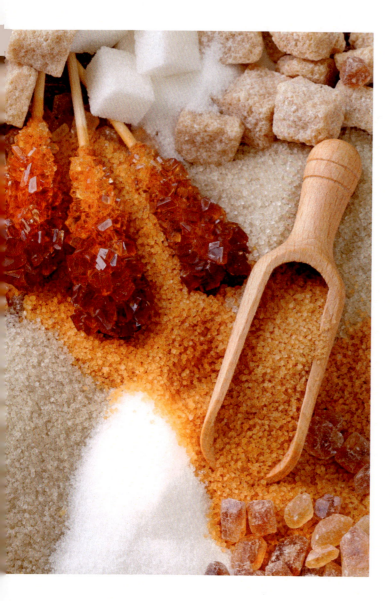

Carbs: What Exactly Are They?

Carbohydrates (carbs) are found in things like starches, grains and foods high in sugar. This includes, but isn't limited to, bread, flour, rice, pasta, beans, potatoes, sugar, syrup, cereals, fruits, bagels and soda.

Carbs are broken down into glucose (a type of sugar) in our bodies for energy. Eating any kinds of carbs spikes blood sugar levels. The spike may happen faster or slower depending on the type of carb (based on the glycemic index), but the spike will still happen.

Blood sugar spikes cause strong insulin releases to combat the spikes. Constant insulin releases result in fat storage and insulin resistance. After many years, this cycle can lead to prediabetes, metabolic syndrome and even type 2 diabetes.[9]

In a world full of sugar, cereal, pasta, burgers, French fries and large sodas, you can see how carbs can easily be overconsumed.

> Almost 1 in 10 adults in the U.S. have type 2 diabetes, nearly 4 times more than 30 years ago.

Where We Are Today

According to the 2014 report by the Centers for Disease Control and Prevention (CDC), more than 1 in 3 adults in the U.S. (86 million people) have prediabetes, a condition in which blood glucose is always high and commonly leads to type 2 diabetes and many other medical problems.[10]

Today, almost 1 in 10 people in the U.S. have type 2 diabetes compared to almost 1 in 40 in 1980.

Fat has been blamed as the bad guy and carbohydrates have been considered crucial and healthy. Companies have been creating low-fat and fat-free, chemical-laden alternatives of nearly every type of food in existence, yet diabetes and heart disease rates are still increasing.

Fat Is Making a Comeback

Hundreds of studies have been conducted in the past ten years which have been corroborating the same data: that eating healthy fats is not detrimental to health and is, in fact, more beneficial than eating a diet high in carbohydrates.

We're starting to understand that carbs in large quantities are much more harmful than previously thought, while most fats are healthy and essential.

The nutritional landscape is changing. Low-carb and similar dietary groups are growing and a nutritional revolution is beginning. We are beginning to realize the detrimental effects of our relationship with excess sugar and carbs.

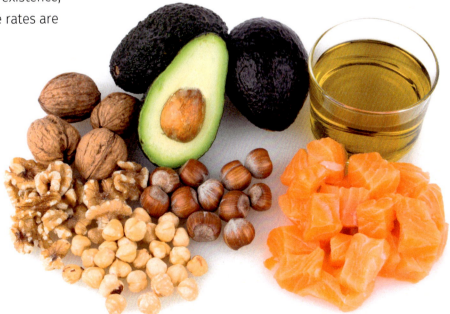

The Basics: Benefits of Going Keto

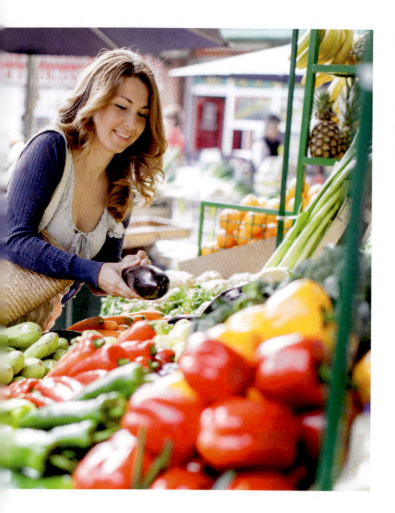

Long-Term Benefits

Studies consistently show that those who eat a low-carb, high-fat diet rather than a high-carb, low-fat diet:

- Lose more weight and body fat[11–17]
- Have better levels of good cholesterol (HDL and large LDL)[18,19]
- Have reduced blood sugar and insulin resistance (commonly reversing prediabetes and type 2 diabetes)[20,21]
- Experience a decrease in appetite[22]
- Have reduced triglyceride levels (fat molecules in the blood that cause heart disease)[19,23]
- Have significant reductions in blood pressure, leading to a reduction in heart disease and stroke[24]

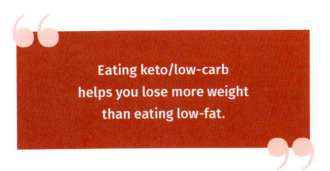

> Eating keto/low-carb helps you lose more weight than eating low-fat.

Day-To-Day Benefits

The keto diet doesn't only provide long-term benefits! When you're on keto, you can expect to:

- Lose body fat
- Have stable energy levels during the day
- Stay satiated after meals longer, with less snacking and overeating

Longer satiation and consistent energy levels are due to the majority of calories coming from fat, which is slower to digest and calorically denser.

Eating low-carb also eliminates blood glucose spikes and crashes. You won't have sudden blood sugar drops leaving you feeling weak and disoriented.

Entering Ketosis

The keto diet's main goal is to keep you in nutritional ketosis all the time. If you're just getting started with your keto diet, you should eat up to 25 grams of carbs per day.

Once you're in ketosis for long enough (about 4 to 8 weeks), you become keto-adapted, or fat-adapted. This is when your glycogen stores in muscles and liver are depleted, you carry less water weight, muscle endurance increases and your overall energy levels are higher.

Once keto-adapted, you can usually eat ≈ 50 grams of net carbs a day to maintain ketosis.

Type 1 Diabetes & Ketoacidosis

If you have type 1 diabetes, consult with your doctor before starting a keto diet. Diabetic ketoacidosis (DKA) is a dangerous condition that can occur if you have type 1 diabetes due to a shortage of insulin.

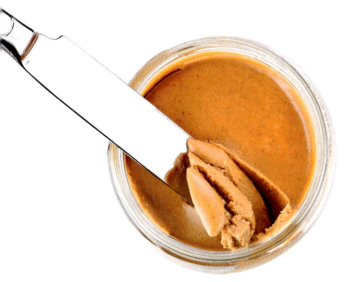

Steering Clear of the Keto Flu

What Is the Keto Flu?

The keto flu happens commonly to keto dieters due to low levels of sodium and electrolytes and has flu-like symptoms including:

- Fatigue
- Headaches
- Cough
- Sniffles
- Irritability
- Nausea

It's important to note that this isn't the real flu! It's called keto flu due to similar symptoms but it is not at all contagious and doesn't actually involve a virus.

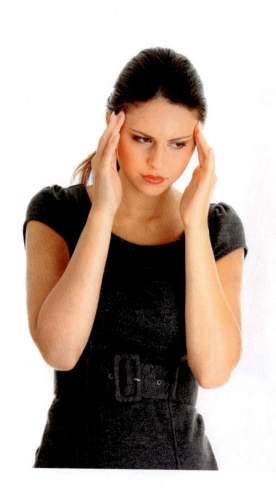

Why Does It Happen?

The main cause of keto flu is your body lacking electrolytes, especially sodium. When starting keto, you cut out lots of processed foods and eat more whole, natural foods. Although this is great, it causes a sudden drop in sodium intake.

> The keto flu can be avoided by consuming enough electrolytes, especially sodium.

In addition, reducing carbs reduces insulin levels, which reduces sodium stored by kidneys.[25]

Between your reduced sodium intake and stored sodium flushed by your kidneys, you end up being low on sodium and other electrolytes.

Ending the Keto Flu

The best way to avoid or end the keto flu is to add more sodium and electrolytes to your diet. Here are the most effective (and tasty) ways to get more sodium:

- Adding more salt to your food
- Drinking soup broth
- Eating plenty of salty foods like bacon and pickled vegetables

Try to eat more sodium as you start the keto diet to prevent the keto flu entirely. If you do catch it, just remember that it'll go away quickly and you'll emerge a fat-burning machine!

Note: *For more information about the keto flu, read our full guide at tasteaholics.com/keto-flu.*

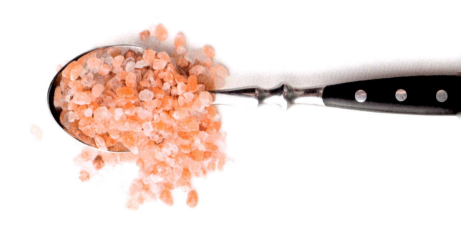

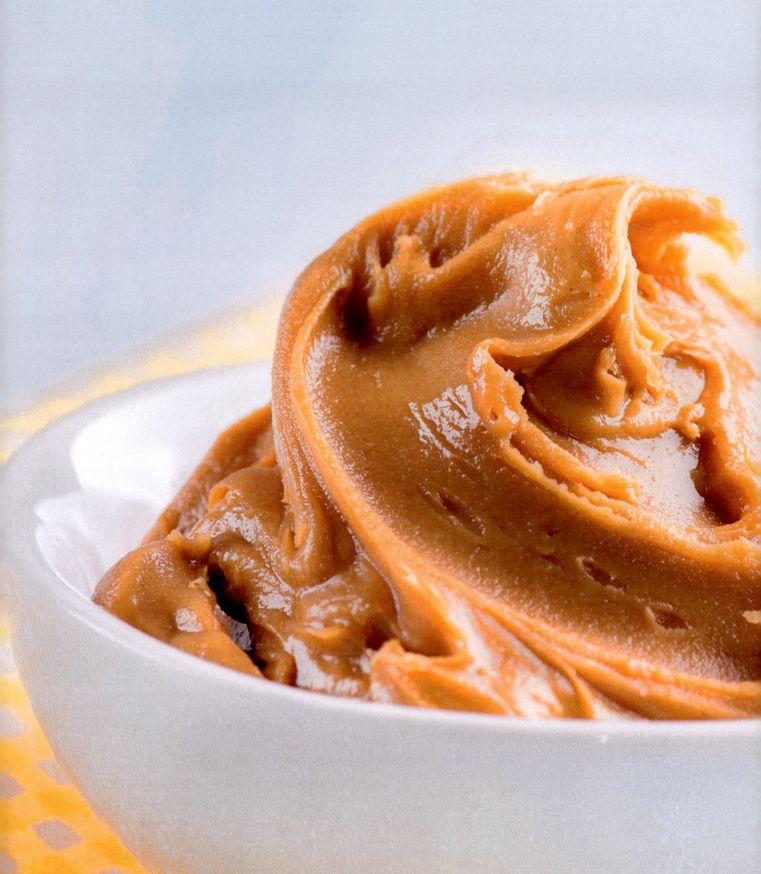

Starting Keto

Part 1 – Out with the Old

Having tempting, unhealthy foods in your home is one of the biggest reasons for failure when starting any diet.

To maximize your chances of success, you need to remove as many triggers as you can. This crucial step will help prevent moments of weakness from ruining all your hard work.

If you aren't living alone, make sure to discuss with your family or housemates before throwing anything out. If some items are simply not yours to throw out, try to compromise and agree on a special location so you can keep them out of sight and out of mind.

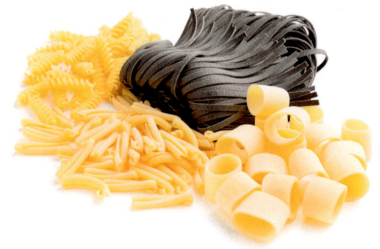

Once your home is free of temptation, eating low-carb is far less difficult and success is that much easier.

Starches and Grains

Get rid of all cereal, pasta, bread, rice, potatoes, corn, oats, quinoa, flour, bagels, rolls, croissants and wraps.

All Sugary Things

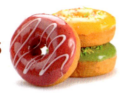

Throw away and forget all refined sugar, fruit juices, desserts, fountain drinks, milk chocolate, pastries, candy bars, etc.

Legumes

Discard or donate any beans, peas, and lentils.

Vegetable & Seed Oils

Stop using any vegetable oils and seed oils like sunflower, safflower, soybean, canola, corn and grapeseed oil. Get rid of trans fats like margarine.

Read Nutrition Labels

Check the nutrition labels on all your products to see if they're high in carbs. There are hidden carbs in the unlikeliest of places (like ketchup and canned soups). Try to avoid buying products with dozens of incomprehensible ingredients. Less is usually healthier.

For example:

Deli ham can have 2 or 3 grams of sugar per slice as well as many added preservatives and nitrites!

Always check the serving sizes against the carb counts. Manufacturers can sometimes recommend inconceivably small serving sizes to seemingly reduce calorie and carb numbers.

At first glance, something may be low in carbs, but a quick comparison to the serving size can reveal the product is mostly sugar. Be diligent!

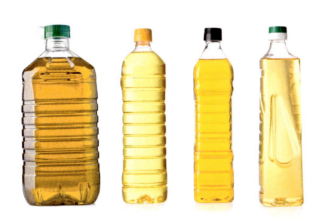

Part 2 – In with the New!

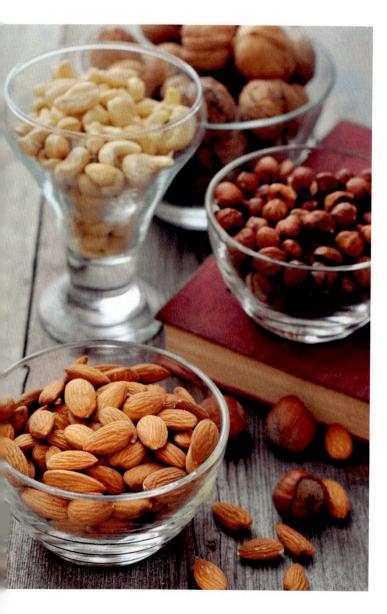

Now that you've cleaned out everything you don't need, it's time to restock your pantry and fridge with delicious and wholesome, keto-friendly foods that will help you lose weight, become healthier, and feel amazing!

General Products to Have

With these basics in your home, you'll always be ready to make healthy, keto-friendly meals.

- Lots of water, coffee, and unsweetened tea
- Stevia and erythritol (sweeteners)
- Condiments like mayonnaise, mustard, pesto, and sriracha
- Broths (beef, chicken, bone)
- Pickles and other fermented foods
- Seeds and nuts (chia seeds, flaxseeds, pecans, almonds, walnuts, macadamias, etc.)

Meat, Fish & Eggs

Just about every type of fresh meat and fish is good for keto including beef, chicken, lamb, pork, salmon, tuna, etc. Eat grass-fed and/or organic meat and wild-caught fish whenever possible.

Eat as many eggs as you like, preferably organic from free-range chicken

Vegetables

Eat plenty of non-starchy veggies including asparagus, mushrooms, broccoli, cucumber, lettuce, onions, peppers, cauliflower, tomatoes, garlic, Brussels sprouts and zucchini.

Dairy

You can eat full-fat dairy like sour cream, heavy (whipping) cream, butter, cheeses and unsweetened yogurt.

Although not dairy, unsweetened almond milk and coconut milk are both good milk substitutes.

Stay away from regular milk, skim milk and sweetened yogurts because they contain a lot of sugar. Avoid all fat-free and low-fat dairy products.

Oils and Fats

Olive oil, avocado oil, butter and bacon fat are great for cooking and consuming. Avocado oil is best for searing due to its very high smoke point (520°F).

Fruits

Berries like strawberries, blueberries, raspberries, etc. are allowed in small amounts. Avocados are great because they're low-carb and very high in fat!

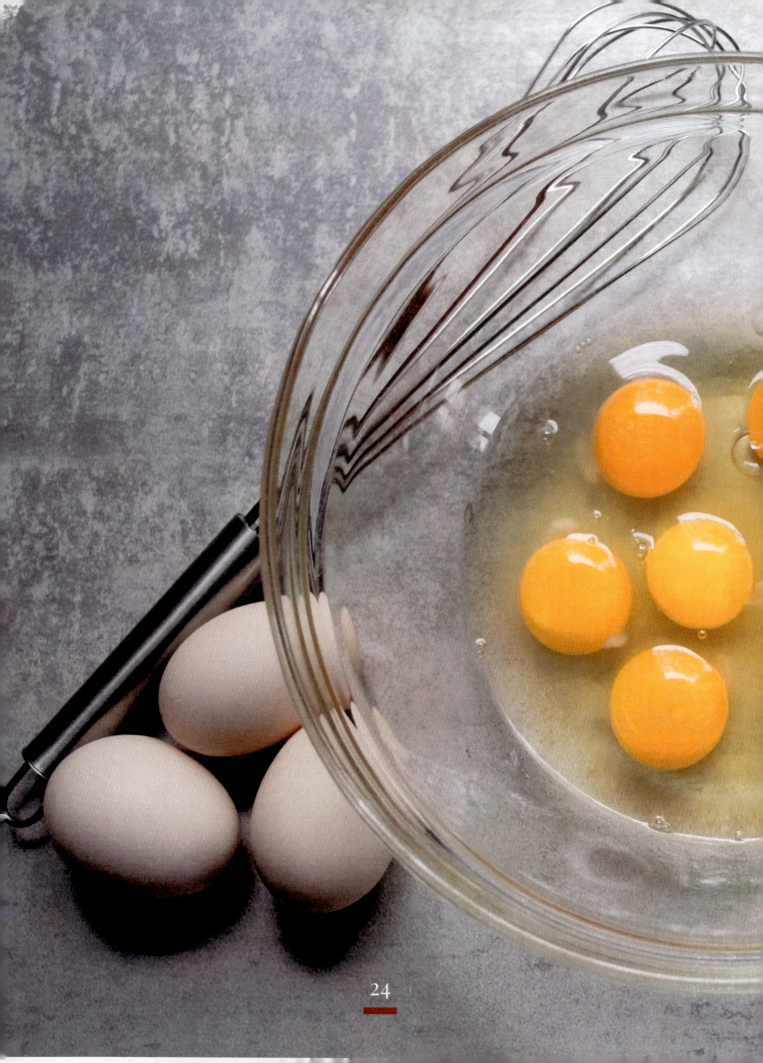

Recipes

Notes

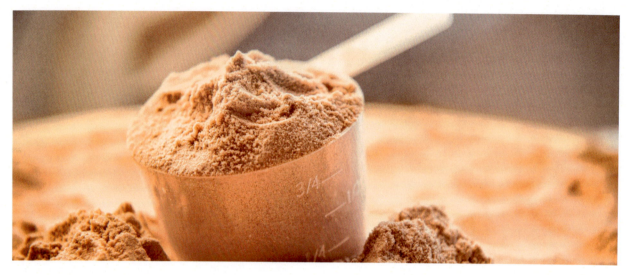

- We use large eggs in all our recipes. If yours are a different size, know that this will affect the nutrition slightly.

- The low-carb protein powder we use is *Isopure* Vanilla and *Isopure* Chocolate.

- Almond milk and coconut milk is always the unsweetened variety.

- Try to find the most natural peanut and almond butter brands you can. The ingredients listed should be, at most, 2 ingredients long.

- If you see the abbreviation "SF" it is short for "sugar-free".
  - For example, "SF Maple Syrup" means we used *Walden Farms* or *Sukrin Gold* syrup, both of which are sugar-free brands.

- A food scale is a must if you're counting calories and macros. Many of our ingredients are listed by weight to provide accurate nutritional data.

- If you don't have stevia, feel free to substitute your favorite sugar-free sweetener like erythritol, xylitol, Splenda, etc. Add a little at a time and work your way up to taste. Stevia is much stronger than these sweeteners and is used in small amounts.

- You can order erythritol online by visiting tasteaholics.com/erythritol.

27

Raspberry Danish Cookies

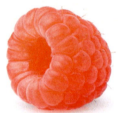

All your favorite things about Danishes turned into bite-sized, baked-to-perfection cookies! Sweet, tart and delightfully dense!

Nutrition

281 calories per 2 cookies | Makes 8 cookies

- 25 grams of fat
- 9 grams of protein
- 4.5 grams of net carbs

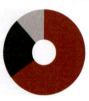

🕒 **Prep Time: 20 mins | Cook Time: 12 mins**

Ingredients

- 4 oz. cream cheese
- 1 large egg
- 6 tbsp. powdered erythritol
- 1 cup almond flour
- 1 oz. raspberries

Instructions

1. To make the dough, blend half the cream cheese, the egg, 4 tablespoons of erythritol and the almond flour with a pinch of salt.
2. To make the Danish filling, beat together the rest of the cream cheese and 1 tablespoon of erythritol in another bowl.
3. In a food processor, pulse 1 tablespoon of erythritol and the raspberries until broken down.
4. Scoop the dough onto a cookie sheet and make a well in each one. Add some of the cream cheese mixture followed by the raspberry mixture.
5. Bake for 12 minutes at 350°F., let cool and enjoy!

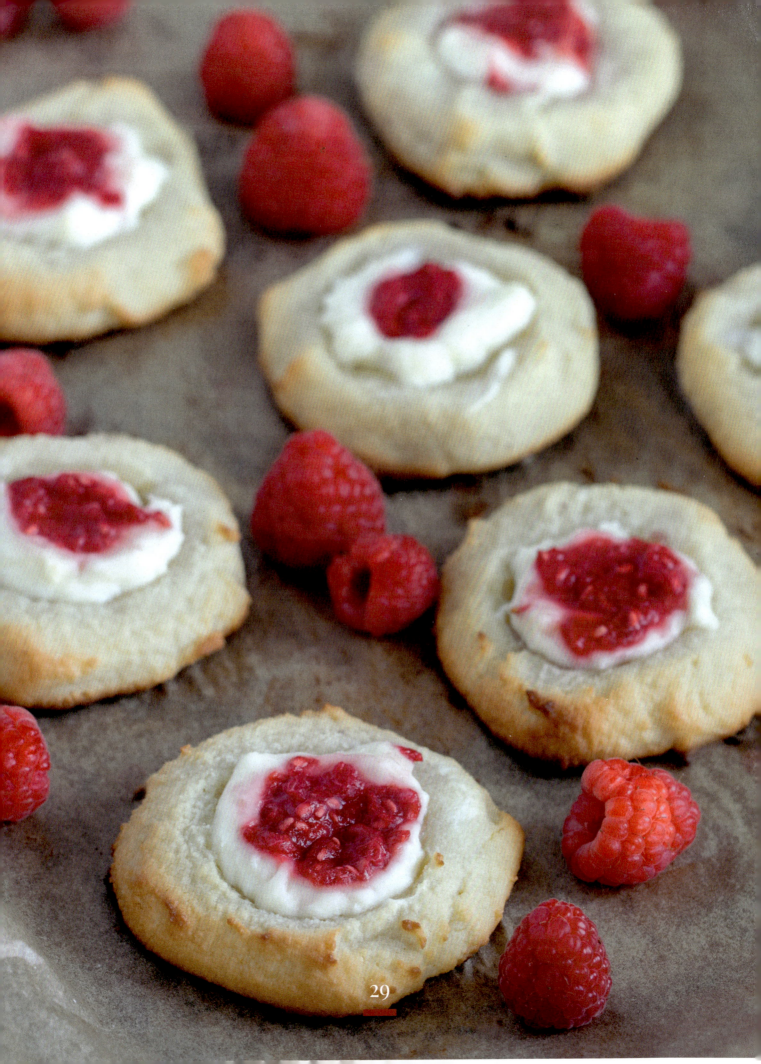

Sugar-Free Nutella

Yes, you read that right: sugar-free *Nutella* can be yours in only 5 ingredients! Our recipe is easy to make and is much healthier than the store-bought stuff.

Nutrition per 2 tbsp.

215 calories per serving | Makes 1 cup

- 20 grams of fat
- 4 grams of protein
- 3 grams of net carbs

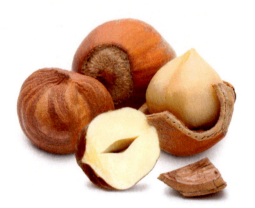

Prep Time: 25 mins | Cook Time: 0 mins

Ingredients

- 2 cups hazelnuts, preferably roasted
- 6 tbsp. cocoa powder
- ½ cup granular erythritol
- 1 tbsp. coconut oil
- ½ cup unsweetened almond milk

Instructions

1. Roast the hazelnuts, if not already roasted, on a baking sheet in a 350°F oven for about 5–10 minutes or until lightly browned.
2. Add the hazelnuts into a food processor and blend until they resemble nut butter.
3. Add in the cocoa powder, erythritol, coconut oil and a pinch of salt. Blend again until fully combined.
4. Add 2 tablespoons of almond milk at a time, blending between each addition. Stop when it reaches a *Nutella*-like consistency. Keep refrigerated and enjoy!

Tip: *Removing the skins off the hazelnuts after toasting will create a silkier finished product, but it's optional!*

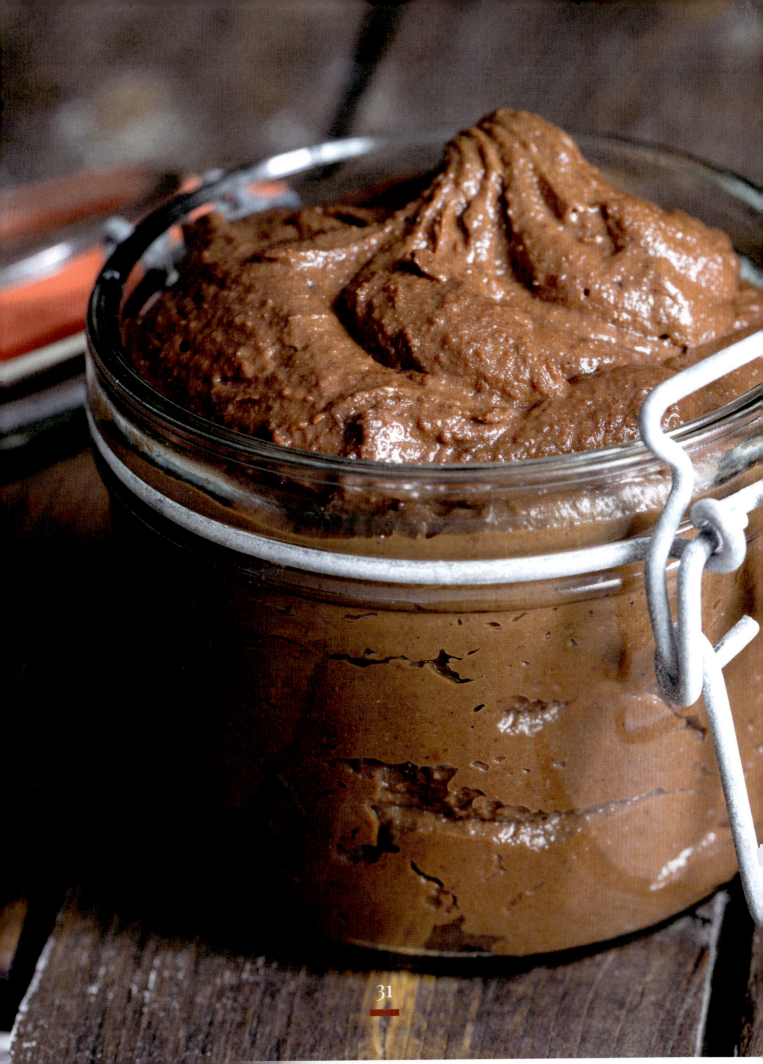

Coconut Cream Pie

The perfect combination of crispy and crunchy paired with smooth and creamy! This coconut cream pie is everything you're dreaming of!

Nutrition

423 calories per serving | Makes 8 slices

- 44 grams of fat
- 3 grams of protein
- 5 grams of net carbs

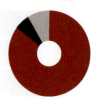

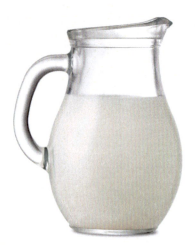

⏱ **Prep Time: 30 mins | Cook Time: 15 mins**

Ingredients

- 200 grams unsweetened flaked coconut
- ¼ cup coconut oil
- ¾ cup powdered erythritol
- ¾ tsp. xanthan gum
- 2 cups heavy cream

Instructions

1. Blend 100 grams of the flaked coconut, coconut oil and ¼ cup erythritol. Press into an 8" round pie pan and bake for 10 minutes at 350°F.
2. Whisk xanthan gum into the heavy cream in a pot on low heat until well incorporated. Then add the powdered erythritol and 50 grams of flaked coconut. Let boil, then let sit for 10 minutes.
3. On a baking sheet, toast 50 grams of flaked coconut for 5 minutes at 350°F.
4. Pour the cream mixture onto the cooled crust.
5. Sprinkle with the toasted flaked coconut and refrigerate for at least 12 hours. Enjoy!

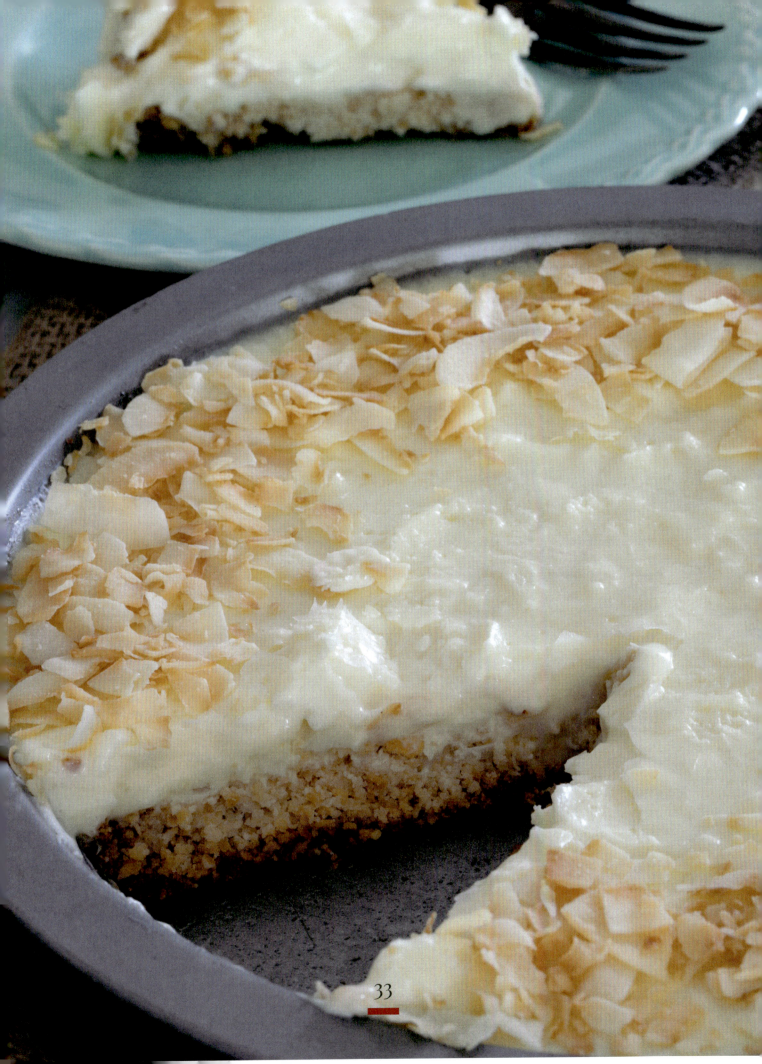

Cheesecake for One

Easier to make than a whole cheesecake but just as delicious! Grab these easy ingredients, some fresh strawberries and get baking.

Nutrition

140 calories per cake | Makes 2 cheesecakes

14 grams of fat
2 grams of protein
2 grams of net carbs

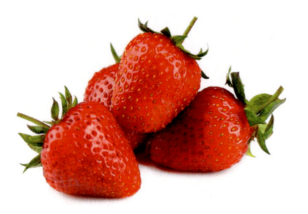

🕐 **Prep Time: 10 mins | Cook Time: 30 mins**

Ingredients

- 6 oz. cream cheese
- 10 drops liquid stevia
- 1 large egg
- 2 tbsp. granular erythritol
- 50 grams strawberries, sliced

Instructions

1. Whip the cream cheese, stevia and a pinch of salt with an electric hand mixer until creamy.
2. Beat an egg in a small bowl and slowly add it to the cream cheese while mixing.
3. Then, add the erythritol and mix to combine.
4. Lightly oil 2 ramekins and divide batter equally. Bake for 30 minutes at 300°F and then chill for about 4 hours or preferably overnight.
5. Top with sliced strawberries and enjoy!

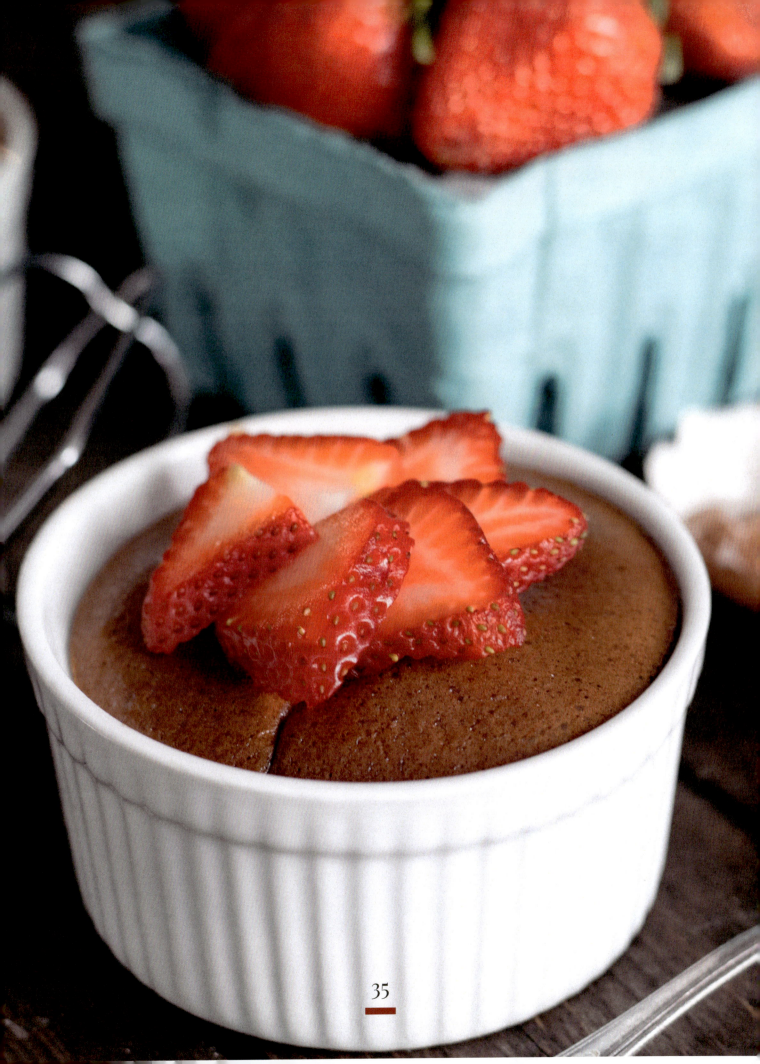

Chocolate Peanut Butter Cups

Your favorite shareable candy can now be made sugar-free! Just 5 easy ingredients and you'll be ready to dig in to peanut buttery goodness.

Nutrition

350 calories per 2 cups | Makes 8 cups

- 29 grams of fat
- 10 grams of protein
- 5 grams of net carbs

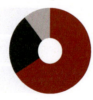

🕒 **Prep Time: 20 mins | Cook Time: 0 mins**

Ingredients

- 4 oz. unsweetened baker's chocolate
- 1 tbsp. coconut oil
- 4 tbsp. powdered erythritol
- 6 tbsp. peanut butter
- 1 pinch of salt

Instructions

1. Melt the chocolate and coconut oil in a double boiler. Add 2 tablespoons of erythritol and salt and stir well to dissolve the erythritol.
2. Equally divide half the chocolate mixture among 8 silicone cupcake molds. Chill until set.
3. Melt the peanut butter in the microwave in 30 second intervals. Add 2 tablespoons of erythritol and stir.
4. Equally divide the peanut butter mixture into the molds over the hardened chocolate. Chill until set.
5. Top with the rest of the chocolate and chill until set. Remove from molds, serve and enjoy!

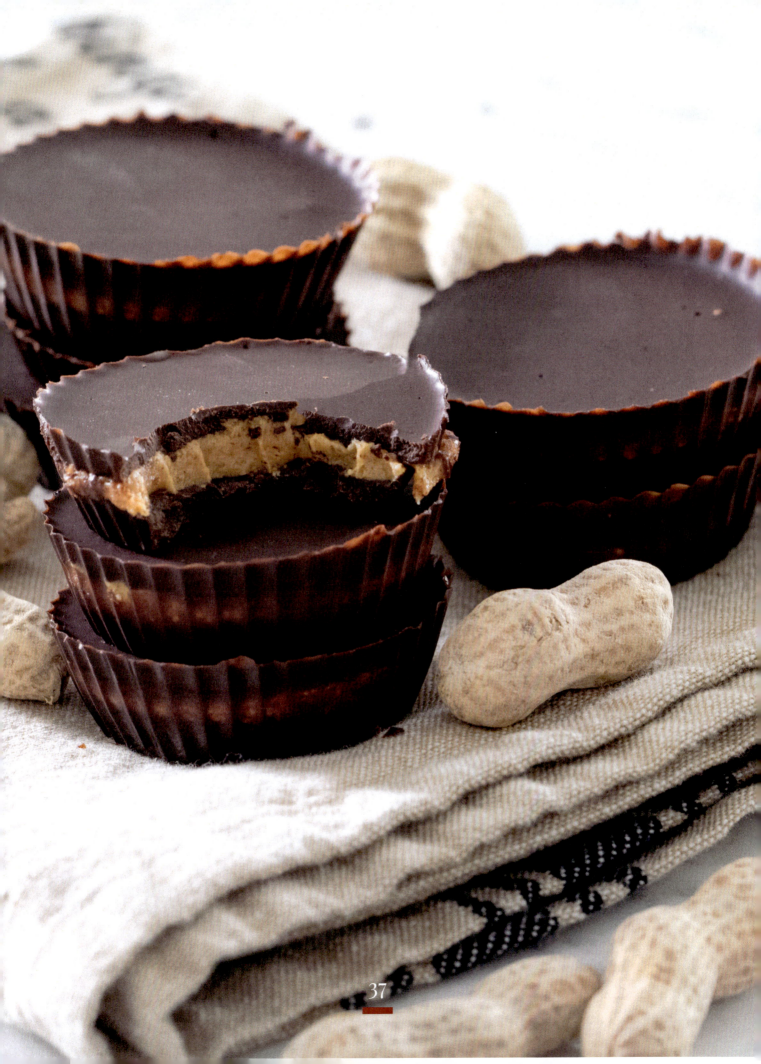

Crazy for Coconut Cake

This sugar-free, dairy-free coconut cake is easy to make and you won't believe how moist and delicate it turns out! A family favorite, for sure.

Nutrition

368 calories per serving | Makes 6 servings

- 36 grams of fat
- 6 grams of protein
- 5 grams of net carbs

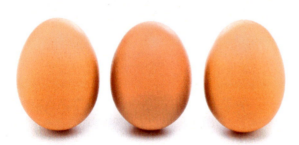

🕐 **Prep Time: 20 mins | Cook Time: 60 mins**

Ingredients

- 2 cups canned unsweetened coconut milk
- ⅓ cup granular erythritol
- 3 large eggs
- ⅓ cup powdered erythritol
- 2 cups unsweetened shredded coconut

Instructions

1. In a pot on medium heat, mix 1 cup of coconut milk with the granular erythritol. Once at a boil, reduce to a simmer for 20 minutes, stirring occasionally.
2. Then, add this mixture to a bowl along with eggs and powdered erythritol and mix to combine well.
3. Add the shredded coconut, the remaining cup of coconut milk and a pinch of salt. Stir well.
4. Bake in a lightly oiled, 8×8" baking dish for 40 minutes at 350°F or until golden.
5. Serve with a sprinkle of shredded coconut and enjoy!

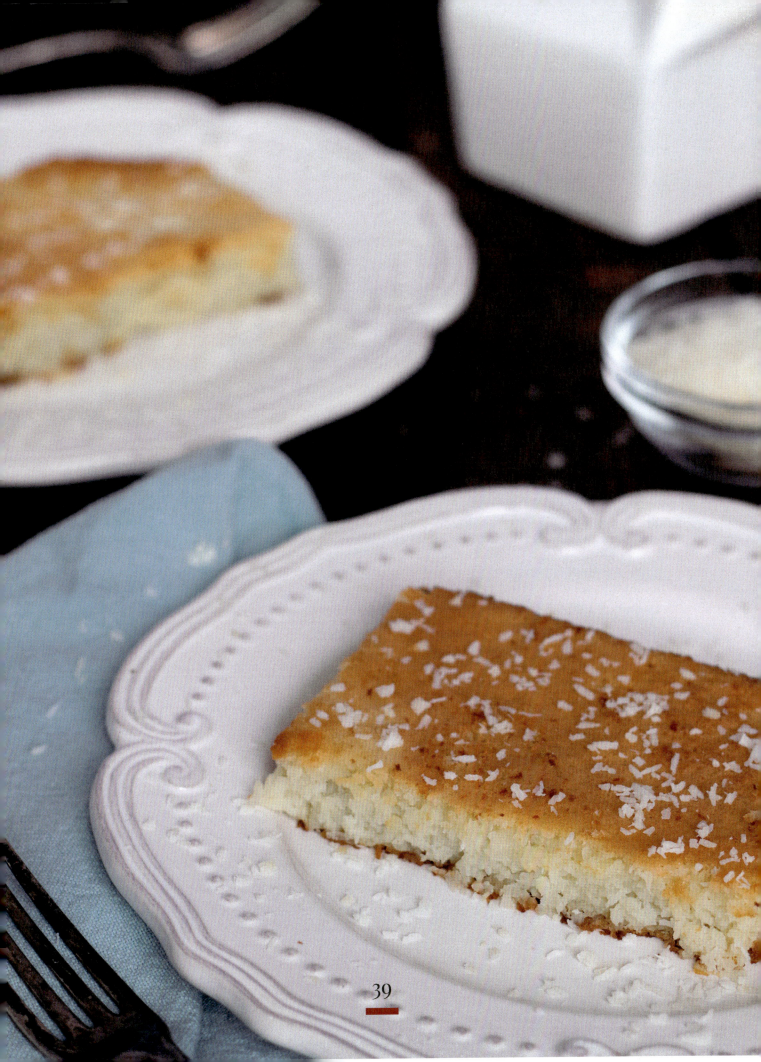

Macadamia Nut Clusters

Sweet, chocolatey and nutty, this dessert has it all. Only 5 ingredients, minimal assembly and absolutely no baking required!

Nutrition

100 calories per cluster | Makes 10 clusters

- 9 grams of fat
- 1 gram of protein
- 1.3 grams of net carbs

Prep Time: 20 mins | Cook Time: 0 mins

Ingredients

- ½ cup heavy cream
- 50 grams unsweetened baker's chocolate
- 15–20 drops liquid stevia
- 10 whole pecans
- 20 macadamia nuts

Instructions

1. Heat the heavy cream on low heat (don't boil it!) and add finely chopped baker's chocolate into it. Stir until fully melted and sweeten with stevia, if desired.
2. Arrange the 1 pecan and 2 macadamias in 10 small piles on a parchment paper-lined baking sheet.
3. Pour or spoon about a teaspoon of the chocolate mixture onto each pile, covering all the nuts to ensure they all stick together.
4. Sprinkle some chopped pecans and sea salt over each cluster and refrigerate until set, about 4 hours.

Tip: *Toast your nuts for deeper flavor!*

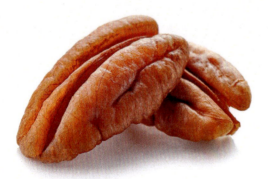

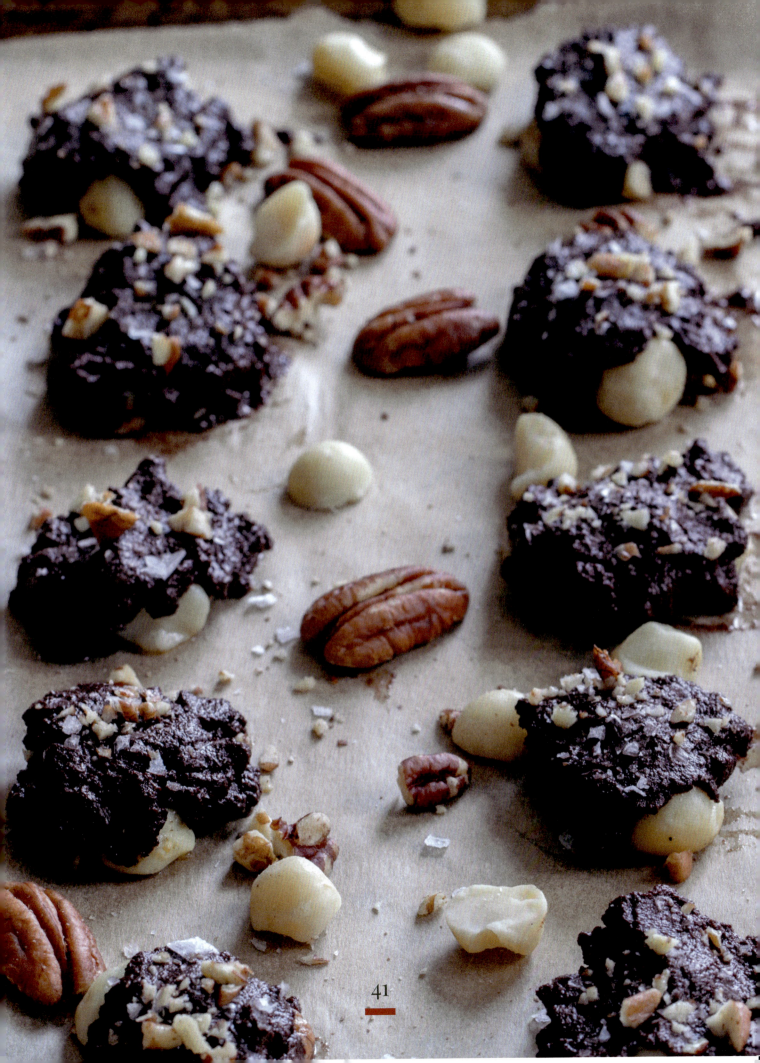

Classic Crème Brûlée

You won't believe the things you can do with erythritol. It even browns and hardens like sugar! Impress everyone with this classic crème brûlée.

Nutrition

475 calories per serving | Makes 2 servings

- 49 grams of fat
- 5 grams of protein
- 4 grams of net carbs

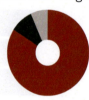

Prep Time: 25 mins | Cook Time: 35 mins

Ingredients

- 4 tbsp. granular erythritol
- 1 cup heavy cream
- 2 large egg yolks
- 1 tsp. vanilla extract
- 1 pinch of salt

Instructions

1. Preheat the oven to 300°F. Add 3 tablespoons of erythritol to heavy cream in a small pot. Heat gently on a low flame until dissolved.
2. Whisk egg yolks, vanilla extract and a pinch of salt until pale and thick. Continue to whisk while SLOWLY adding in the heavy cream to the egg yolks.
3. Place 2 ramekins in a baking dish and pour hot water into the dish until halfway up the ramekins' sides.
4. Pour the crème brûlée batter into the ramekins and bake for 35 minutes.
5. Chill for at least 4 hours. Before serving, sprinkle ½ a tablespoon of erythritol per ramekin on top and broil until caramelized.

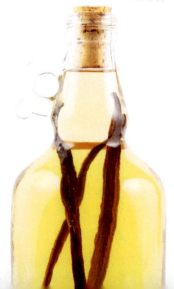

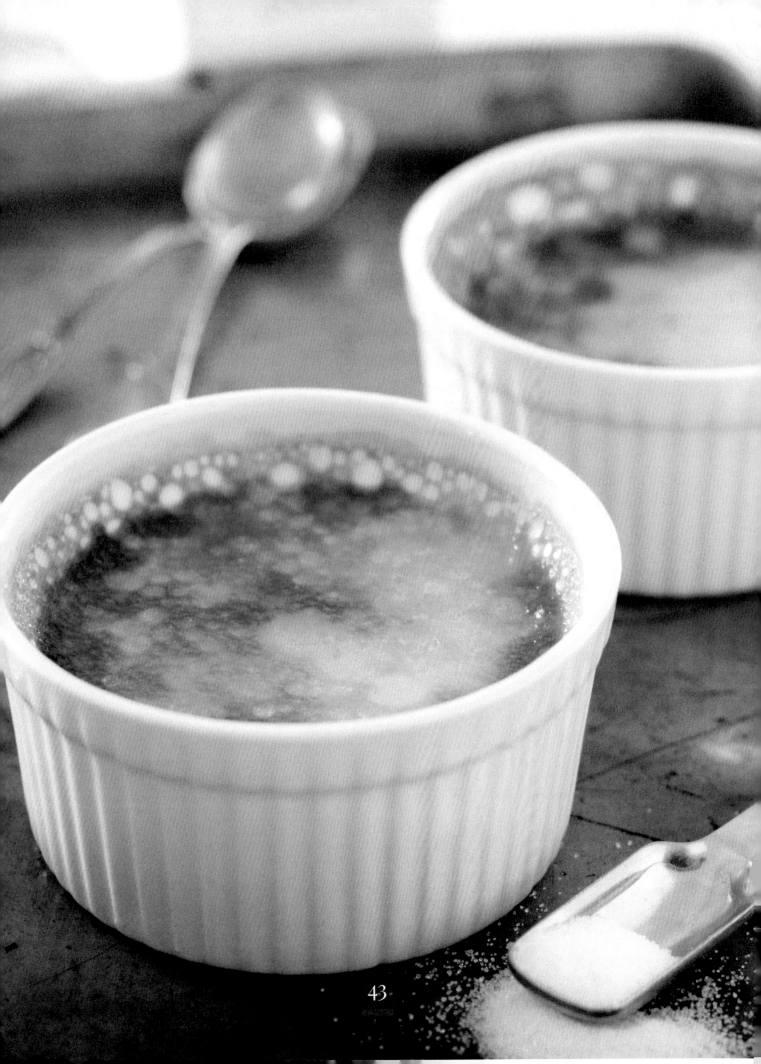

Double Chocolate Mousse

Two kinds of chocolate are better than one! Layer our double chocolate mousse into a container of your choice and enjoy its creaminess!

Nutrition

469 calories per serving | Makes 2 servings

- 45 grams of fat
- 7 grams of protein
- 5 grams of net carbs

🕒 **Prep Time: 25 mins | Cook Time: 0 mins**

Ingredients

- 1 oz. sugar-free chocolate chips
- 1 cup heavy cream
- 4 oz. cream cheese
- ¼ cup powdered erythritol
- 2 tbsp. cocoa powder

Instructions

1. Melt the chocolate chips on very low heat in a pan with ¼ cup of heavy cream.
2. In a bowl, beat the cream cheese and erythritol. Then, add in the melted chocolate chips, cocoa powder and a pinch of salt. Beat well until fully incorporated.
3. In another bowl, beat the remaining ¾ cup of heavy cream until whipped.
4. Into 2 glass serving glasses, layer: chocolate, cream, chocolate, cream and top with more chocolate chips and/or chocolate shavings.

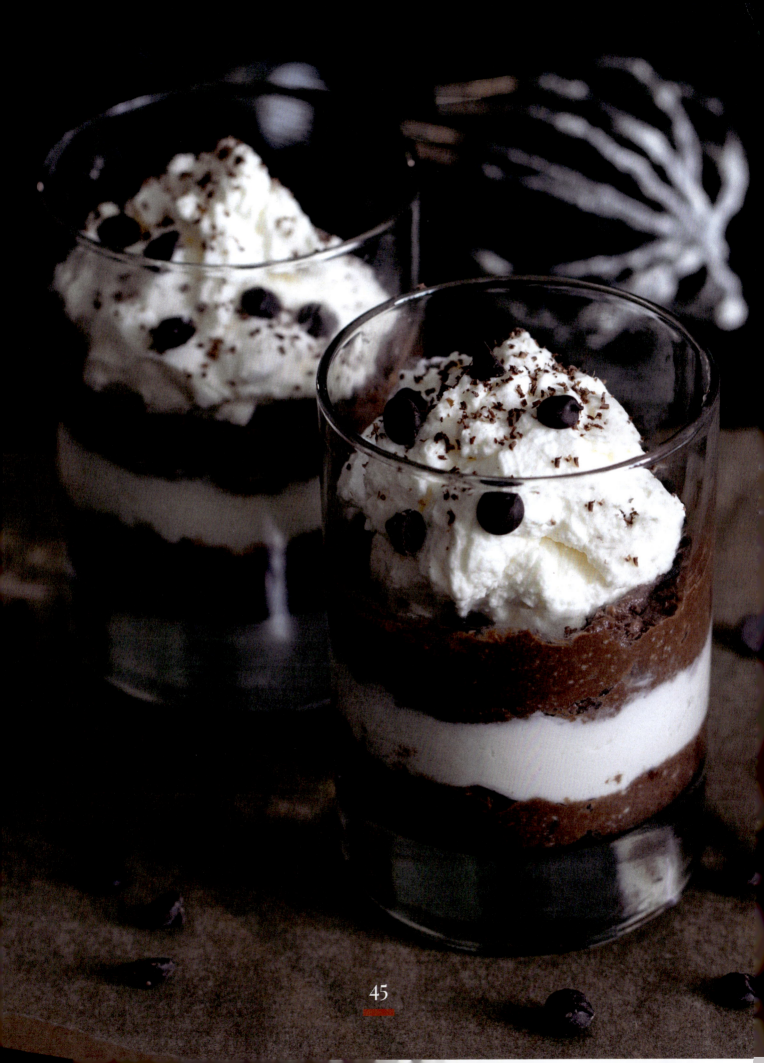

Lemon Dream Bars

You and your guests will be left satisfied after these dense, wonderful lemon dream bars! Finish them off with lemon and a sprinkle of erythritol.

Nutrition

272 calories per serving | Makes 8 servings

- 26 grams of fat
- 8 grams of protein
- 4 grams of net carbs

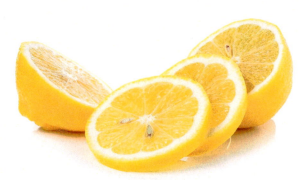

Prep Time: 20 mins | Cook Time: 45 mins

Ingredients

- ½ cup unsalted butter, melted
- 1¾ cups almond flour
- 1 cup powdered erythritol
- 3 medium lemons
- 3 large eggs

Instructions

1. Mix butter, 1 cup almond flour, ¼ cup erythritol and a pinch of salt. Press evenly into an 8×8" parchment paper-lined baking dish. Bake for 20 minutes at 350°F. Then let cool for 10 minutes.
2. Into a bowl, zest one of the lemons, then juice all 3 lemons, add in the eggs, ¾ cup erythritol, ¾ cup almond flour and a pinch of salt. Mix well to make the bars' filling.
3. Pour the filling onto the cooled crust and bake for 25 minutes.
4. Serve with lemon slices and a sprinkle of powdered erythritol.

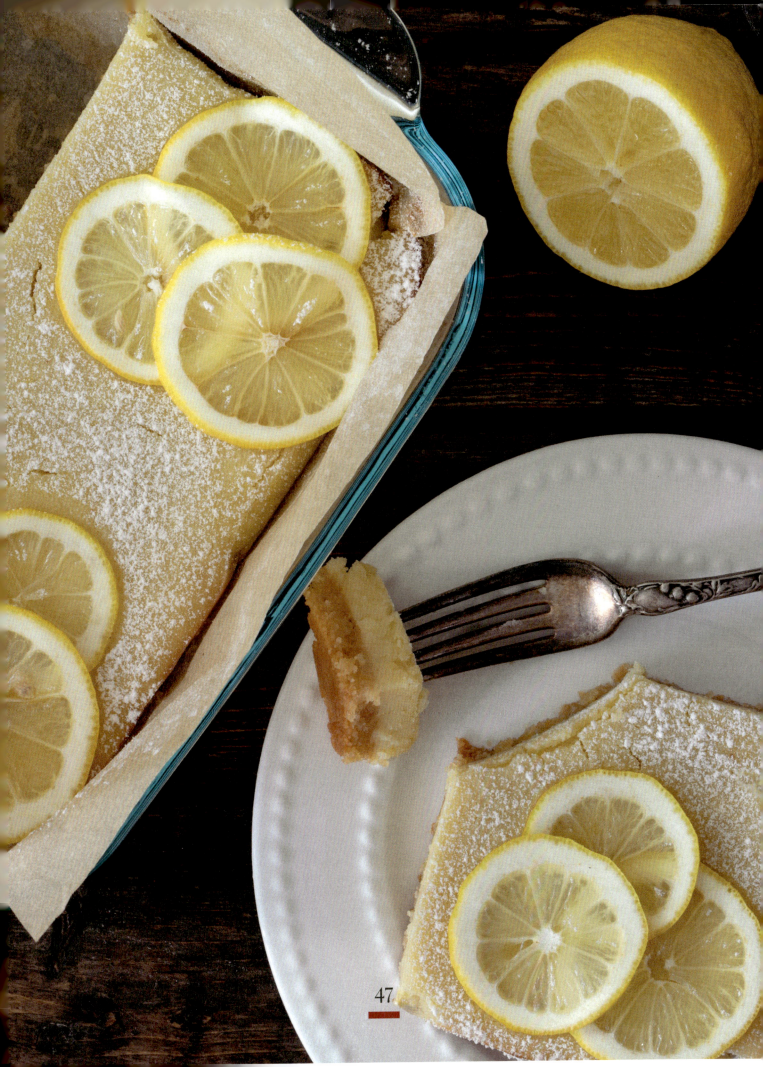

Avocado Chocolate Mousse

Don't knock it 'til you've tried it! Putting avocado into desserts gives them a silky, creamy texture without adding too many extra carbs!

Nutrition

290 calories per serving | Makes 2 servings

- 25 grams of fat
- 6 grams of protein
- 3 grams of net carbs

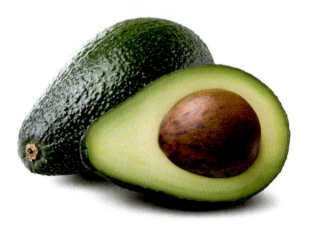

Prep Time: 10 mins | Cook Time: 0 mins

Ingredients

- 300 grams avocado (about 2 medium fruit)
- 6 tsp. cocoa powder
- 3 tbsp. granular erythritol
- 1 tsp. vanilla extract
- 2 tbsp. unsweetened almond milk

Instructions

1. Peel and core the 2 avocados.
2. Add them, along with the rest of the ingredients and a pinch of salt into a food processor and blend until smooth and creamy.
3. Divide into two serving dishes and enjoy!

Tip: *A pinch of cayenne pepper makes this a spiced treat and can mask the flavor of the avocado even more!*

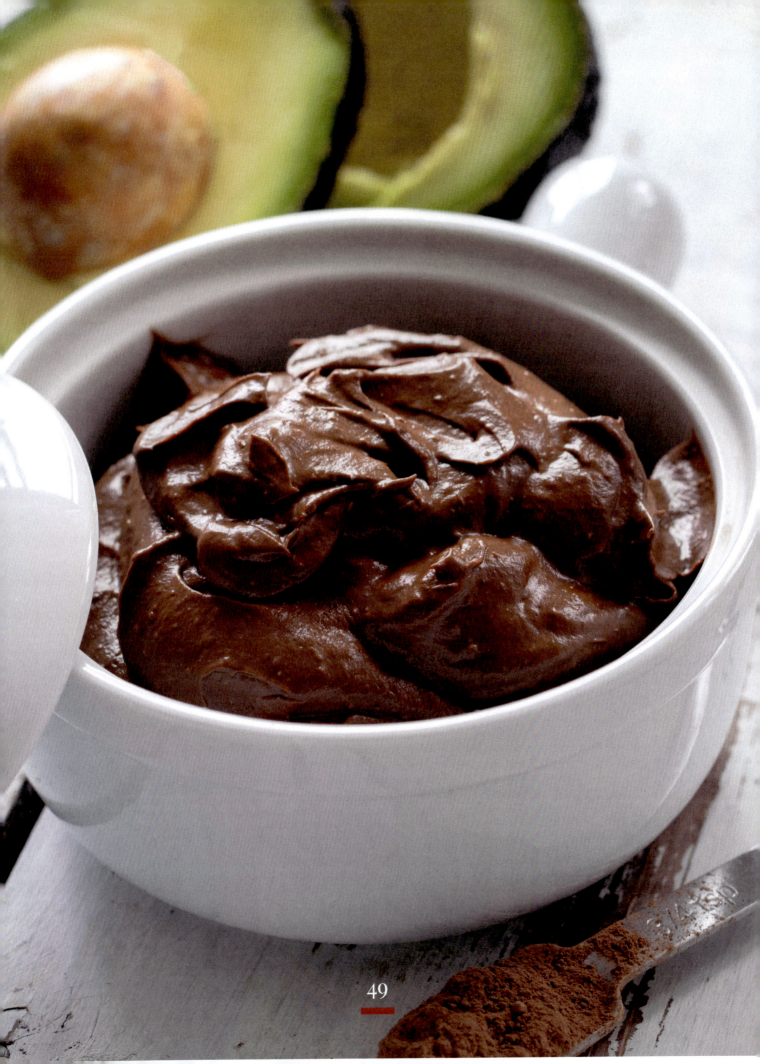

Stracciatella Gelato

Stracciatella gelato is the Italian phrase for chocolate chip ice cream! Feel like you're in Italy for a moment with every bite (or lick).

Nutrition

440 calories per serving | Makes 4 servings

- 43 grams of fat
- 5 grams of protein
- 5 grams of net carbs

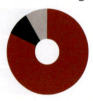

🕐 **Prep Time: 30 mins | Cook Time: 0 mins**

Ingredients

- ⅔ cup granular erythritol
- 1 tsp. vanilla extract
- 1¾ cups heavy cream
- 3 large egg yolks
- ⅓ cup sugar-free chocolate chips

Instructions

1. Add erythritol, vanilla extract and a pinch of salt to the heavy cream in a pot and heat gently until dissolved.
2. Whisk the egg yolks in a bowl. Slowly add 1–2 ladles of the hot cream while whisking to temper the eggs so they don't cook.
3. Pour the egg yolk mixture into the pot and gently heat until the whole thing can coat the back of a spoon. Then let cool *completely*.
4. Pour the batter into the (frozen overnight) drum of an ice cream maker and let it churn according to instructions. Add chocolate chips in the last 5 minutes. Chill in the freezer for a minimum of 4 hours and serve!

Tip: Add 1 tablespoon of vodka in step 3 to keep the ice cream soft after freezing.

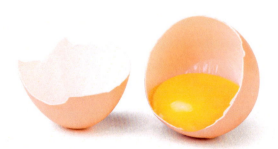

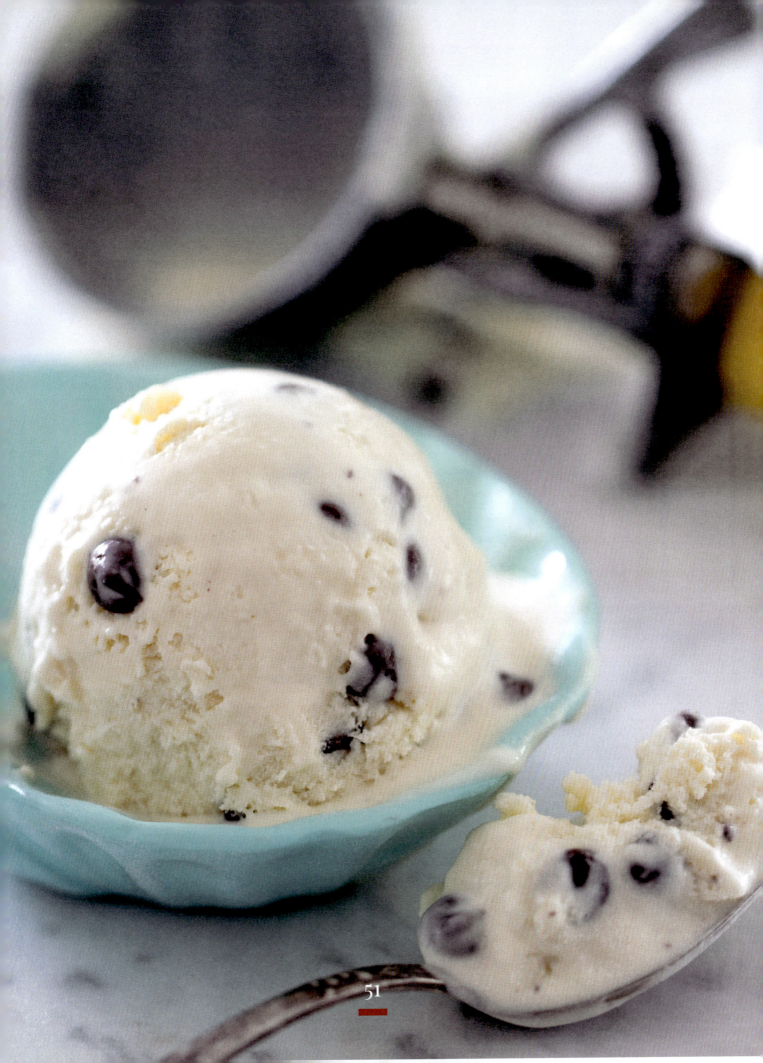

Almond Fudge Brownies

These almond butter brownies are full of fat and fiber. You'll love them with a scoop of your favorite low-carb ice cream!

Nutrition

153 calories per brownie | Makes 12 brownies

- 14 grams of fat
- 8 grams of protein
- 3 grams of net carbs

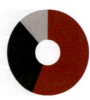

🕒 **Prep Time: 15 mins | Cook Time: 11 mins**

Ingredients

- 1 cup almond butter
- ¾ cup powdered erythritol
- 3 large eggs
- 10 tbsp. cocoa powder
- ½ tsp. baking powder

Instructions

1. Use a food processor to blend together the almond butter and erythritol.
2. Then, add in the eggs, cocoa powder, baking powder and a pinch of salt.
3. Transfer the batter into a greased 9×9" baking pan and smooth the top with a spatula.
4. Bake for 11 minutes at 325°F. Cool completely to firm up before cutting and enjoying.

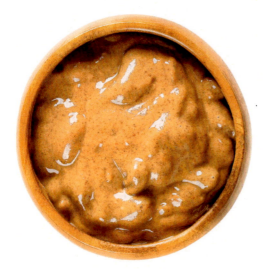

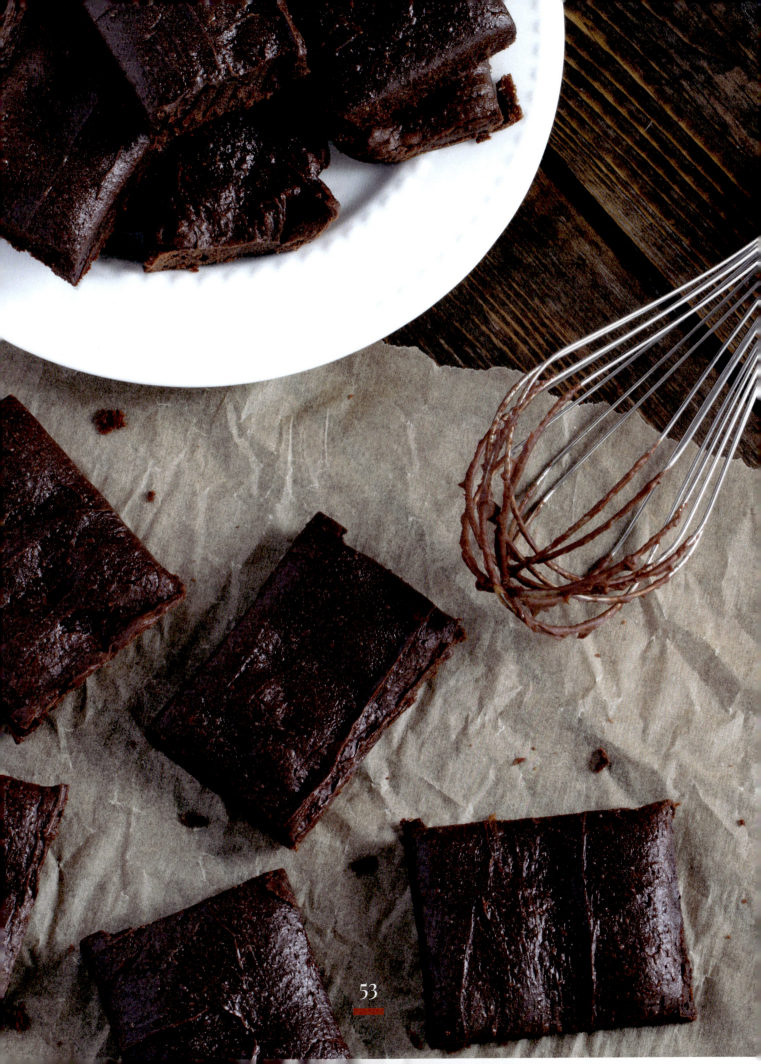

Strawberries & Cream Pancakes

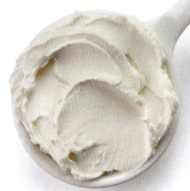

A simple twist on cream cheese pancakes makes this recipe moist and absolutely bursting with flavor! A griddle is a must with these pancakes.

Nutrition

180 calories per 3 pancakes | Makes 6 pancakes

- 14 grams of fat
- 8.5 grams of protein
- 3 grams of net carbs

🕒 **Prep Time: 15 mins | Cook Time: 10 mins**

Ingredients

- 2 large eggs, separated
- ½ tsp. baking powder
- 50 grams strawberries, minced
- 2 oz. cream cheese
- 10 drops liquid stevia

Instructions

1. Beat the egg whites with an electric hand mixer until foamy, then add in the baking powder. Beat until stiff peaks form.
2. Beat the egg yolks, minced strawberries, 1 oz. of cream cheese and stevia until smooth and pale. Combine with the egg whites very gently. Do not deflate the stiff egg whites!
3. Cube the remaining cream cheese and gently mix it into the pancake batter.
4. Ladle ¼ cup of batter at a time onto a griddle on low heat and cook for about 5–7 minutes or until almost fully cooked.
5. *Very* gently, flip and cook for another 1–2 minutes.

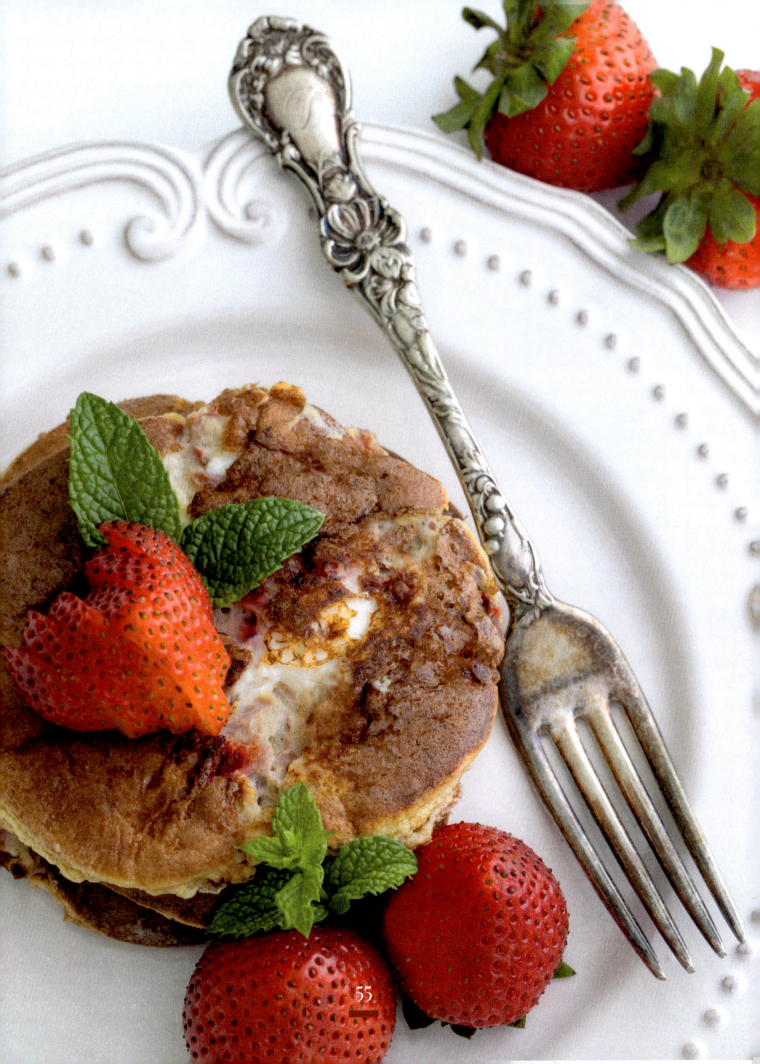

Cinnamon Mug Cake

Cinnamon is a great aromatic spice to add to cakes to make it feel like a cozy autumn's day. We love it in our low-carb desserts!

Nutrition

355 calories | Makes 1 cake

- 32 grams of fat
- 12 grams of protein
- 4 grams of net carbs

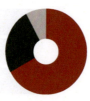

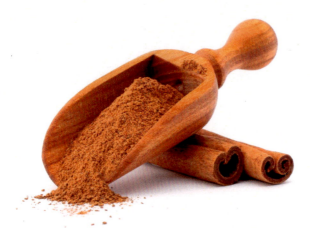

🕐 **Prep Time: 8 mins | Cook Time: 10 mins**

Ingredients

- ¼ cup almond flour
- 2.5 tbsp. granular erythritol
- ½ tsp. ground cinnamon
- 1 large egg
- 1 tbsp. coconut oil

Instructions

1. Combine almond flour, erythritol, cinnamon and a pinch of salt in a bowl.
2. Then, add the egg and coconut oil. Mix well.
3. Lightly oil a ramekin and add the mug cake batter. Bake at 350°F for about 10 minutes or microwave for 1 minute.
4. Enjoy with a drizzle of sugar-free maple syrup (optional, see p. 26).

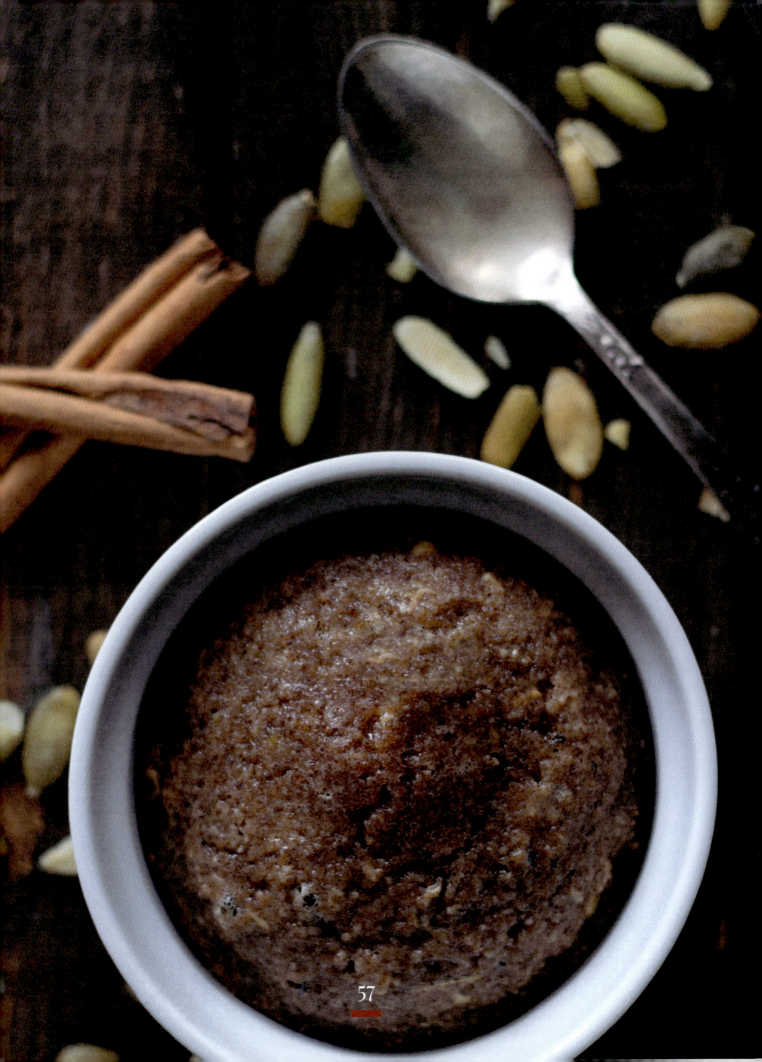

Cookie Dough Mousse

Our cookie dough mousse recipe is perfect for when that hankering for cookie dough arises! It's completely egg-free, so go ahead, munch away!

Nutrition

388 calories per serving | Makes 2 servings

- 37 grams of fat
- 6 grams of protein
- 5 grams of net carbs

🕐 **Prep Time: 10 mins | Cook Time: 0 mins**

Ingredients

- 2 tbsp. unsalted butter
- 4 oz. cream cheese
- 1.5 tsp. vanilla extract
- ¼ cup powdered erythritol
- ¼ cup sugar-free chocolate chips

Instructions

1. Melt the butter on very low heat until golden brown. Do not let it burn!
2. With an electric hand mixer, beat together the cream cheese, vanilla extract, erythritol, browned butter and a pinch of salt.
3. When smooth and combined, fold in the chocolate chips with a spatula.
4. Chill for an hour and enjoy!

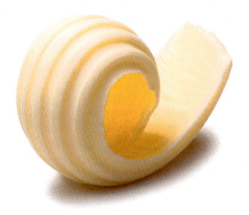

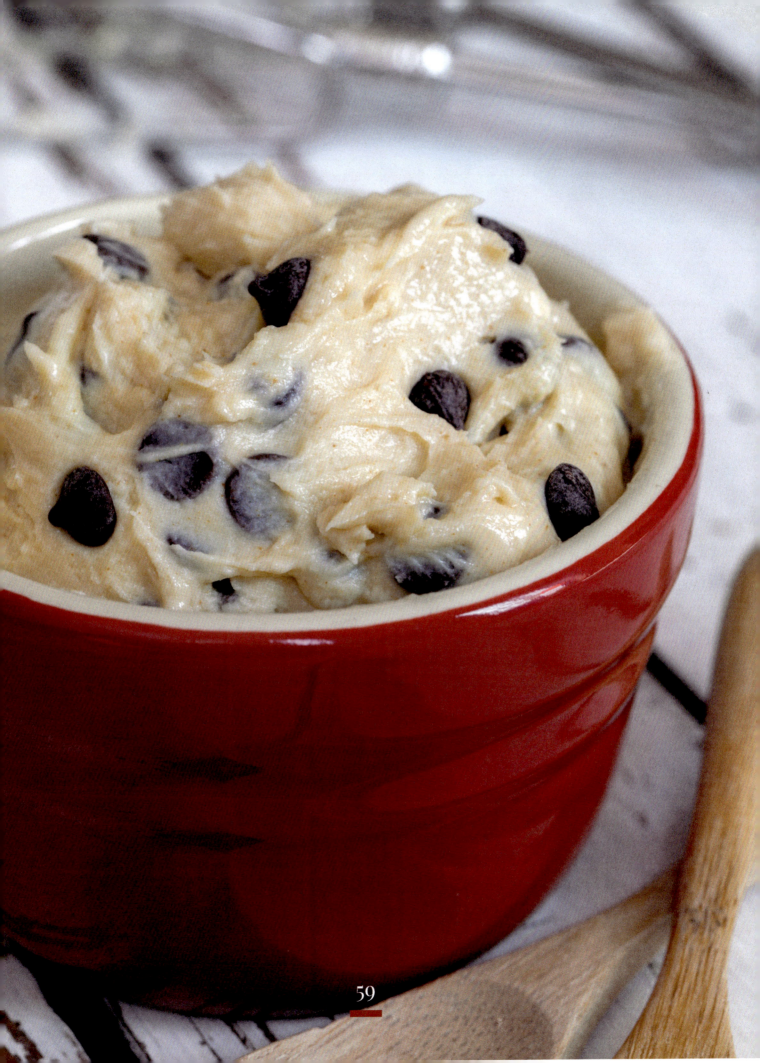

Creamy Coconut Fudge

Light, creamy and uber fudgy! These creamy coconut fudge bites are full of deep, chocolatey flavor with hints of coconut!

Nutrition

220 calories per 2 squares | Makes 16 squares

- 22 grams of fat
- 3 grams of protein
- 3 grams of net carbs

🕐 **Prep Time: 10 mins | Cook Time: 0 mins**

Ingredients

- 8 oz. cream cheese
- 8 tbsp. coconut oil
- ½ cup cocoa powder
- ½ cup granular erythritol
- ¼ cup unsweetened flaked coconut

Instructions

1. Combine cream cheese, coconut oil, cocoa powder, erythritol and a pinch of salt in a pot on medium heat. Heat and stir until all melted.
2. To get rid of any clumps and make everything extra creamy, beat the mixture with an electric hand mixer.
3. Pour the mixture into a parchment paper-lined, 8×8" baking dish and spread to flatten. Sprinkle the top with unsweetened, toasted coconut flakes.
4. Chill overnight and then cut into 16 squares. Enjoy!

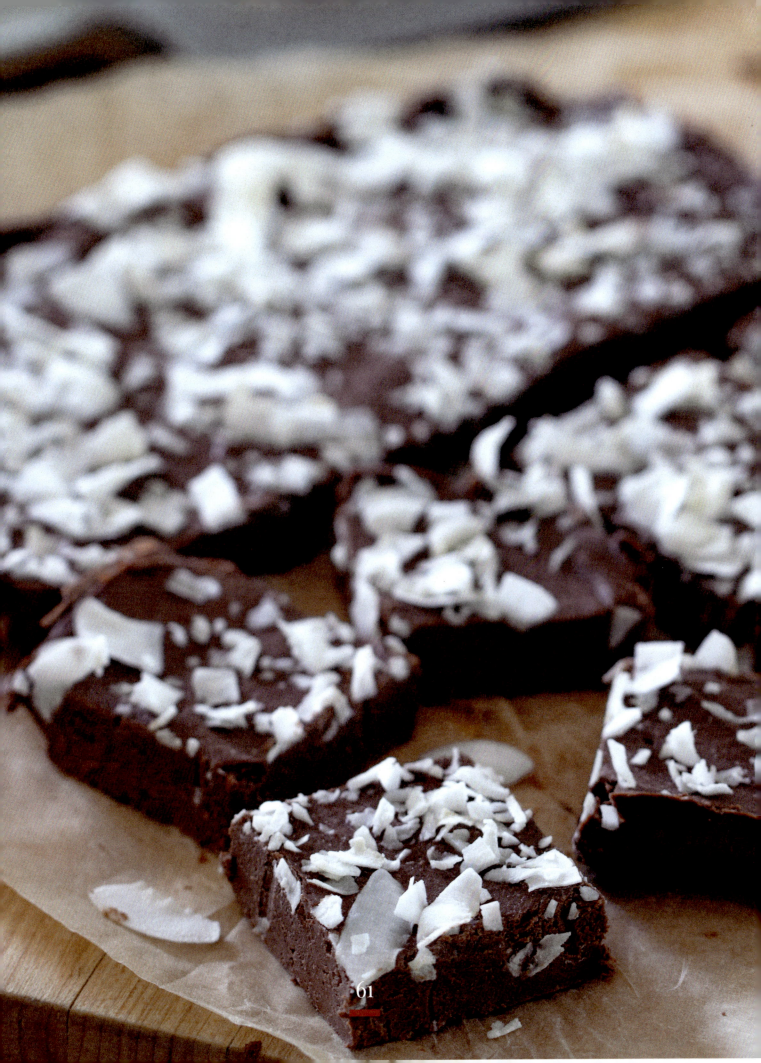

Banana Pudding

Thought you could never enjoy banana in your desserts? Think again! A vial of banana extract will add some delightfully fruity flavor to recipes.

Nutrition

455 calories per serving | Makes 1 cup

- 45 grams of fat
- 3 grams of protein
- 4.5 grams of net carbs

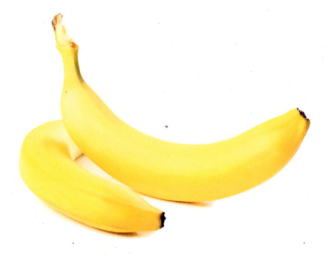

🕐 **Prep Time: 10 mins | Cook Time: 0 mins**

Ingredients

- ½ cup heavy cream
- 1 large egg yolk
- 3 tbsp. powdered erythritol
- ½ tsp. xanthan gum
- ½ tsp. banana extract

Instructions

1. In a double boiler, combine the heavy cream, egg yolk and erythritol. Whisk constantly until the mixture thickens and erythritol dissolves.
2. Add the xanthan gum and whisk until thickened even more. The mixture should be able to coat the back of a spoon.
3. Add in the banana extract and a pinch of salt. Stir and transfer to a small serving dish. Cover with plastic wrap so that it touches the surface of the pudding.
4. Refrigerate for about 4 hours and enjoy!

Tip: *Try this recipe with any flavor extracts of your choice!*

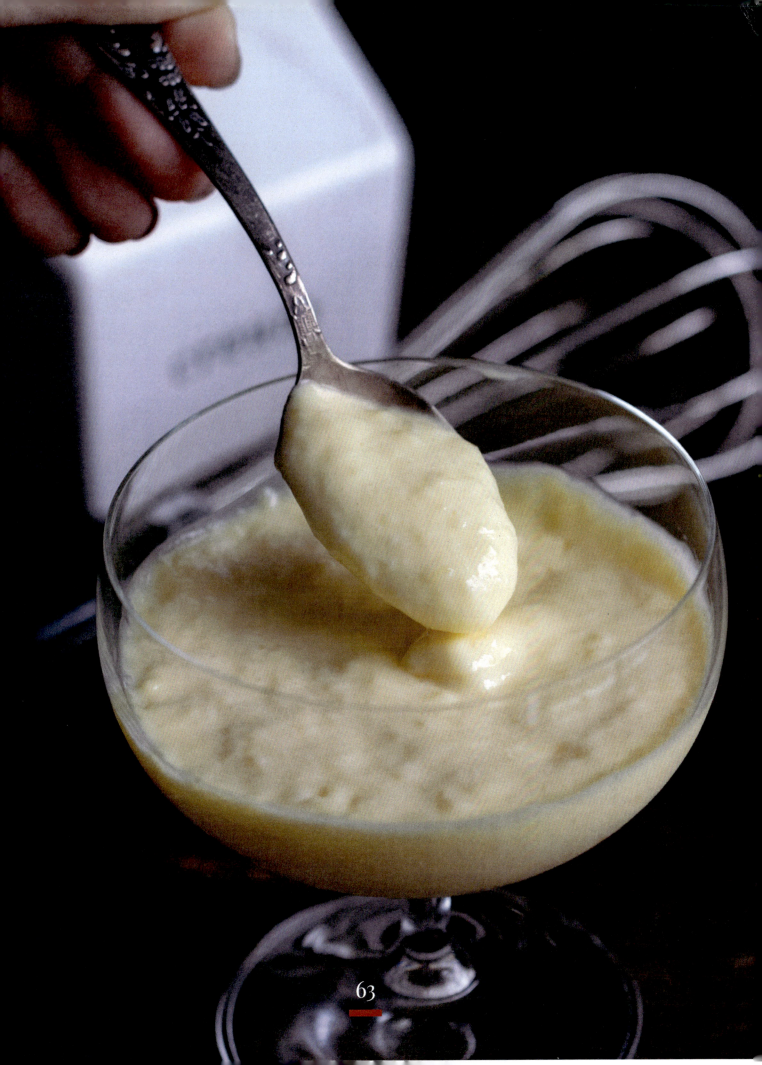

Sea Salt Chocolate Truffles

These truffles were meant to please a crowd. The next time you've got a hungry family coming over, make this recipe and watch them love it!

Nutrition

110 calories per truffle | Makes 10 truffles

- 10 grams of fat
- 1.5 grams of protein
- 1 gram of net carbs

🕐 **Prep Time: 25 mins | Cook Time: 0 mins**

Ingredients

- ½ cup heavy cream
- 4 oz. unsweetened baker's chocolate
- 2 tbsp. unsalted butter
- ½ cup granular erythritol
- 1 tsp. sea salt flakes

Instructions

1. In a double boiler, heat the heavy cream until hot.
2. Cut the chocolate into very small pieces and add them to the hot heavy cream. Stir until melted.
3. Take the bowl off the heat and stir in the butter. Add the erythritol, stir, and refrigerate for 1 hour.
4. Using a cookie scoop, scoop 1-inch balls, rounding them with your lightly oiled hands. Place them on a parchment paper-lined plate and sprinkle each with some sea salt flakes.
5. Refrigerate until set, about 1-2 hours, then enjoy!

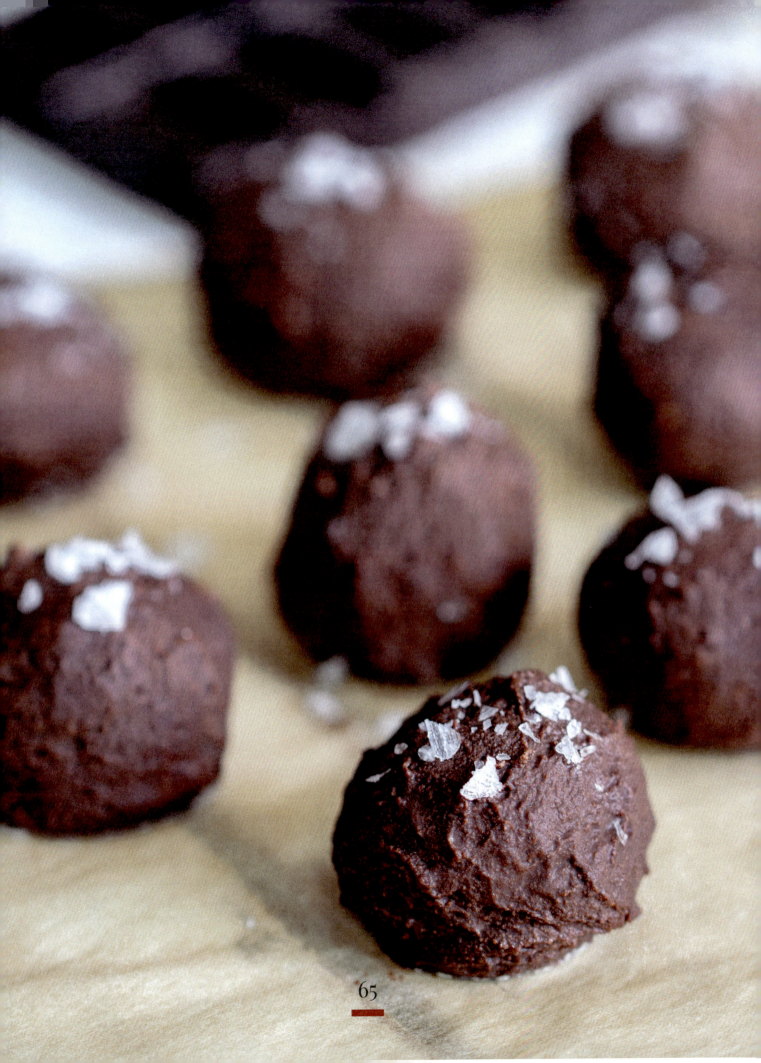

Double Lemon Jell-O Cake

So light and fluffy, this double lemon Jell-O cake is a dream come true! Each bite is its own little piece of heaven right in your mouth.

Nutrition

408 calories per serving | Makes 4 servings

- 41 grams of fat
- 7 grams of protein
- 4 grams of net carbs

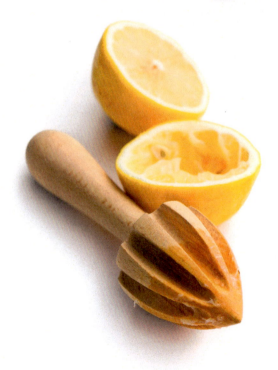

🕐 **Prep Time: 15 mins | Cook Time: 15 mins**

Ingredients

- 100 grams pecans
- 1 tbsp. unsalted butter, melted
- 8.5 grams sugar-free lemon Jell-O
- 8 oz. cream cheese
- 2 tbsp. fresh lemon juice

Instructions

1. Make the crust by blending together the pecans, melted butter and a pinch of salt in a food processor. Do not overblend into nut butter, just until it's very finely crushed.
2. Press the crust into a 6×6" baking dish. Bake at 350°F for 15 minutes. It should be dry to the touch. After, let it cool for 15 minutes.
3. Whisk the Jell-O powder with 1 cup of boiling water, then add cream cheese and lemon juice. Whisk until smooth.
4. Pour in the Jell-O cream cheese mixture and let chill in the refrigerator overnight. Enjoy!

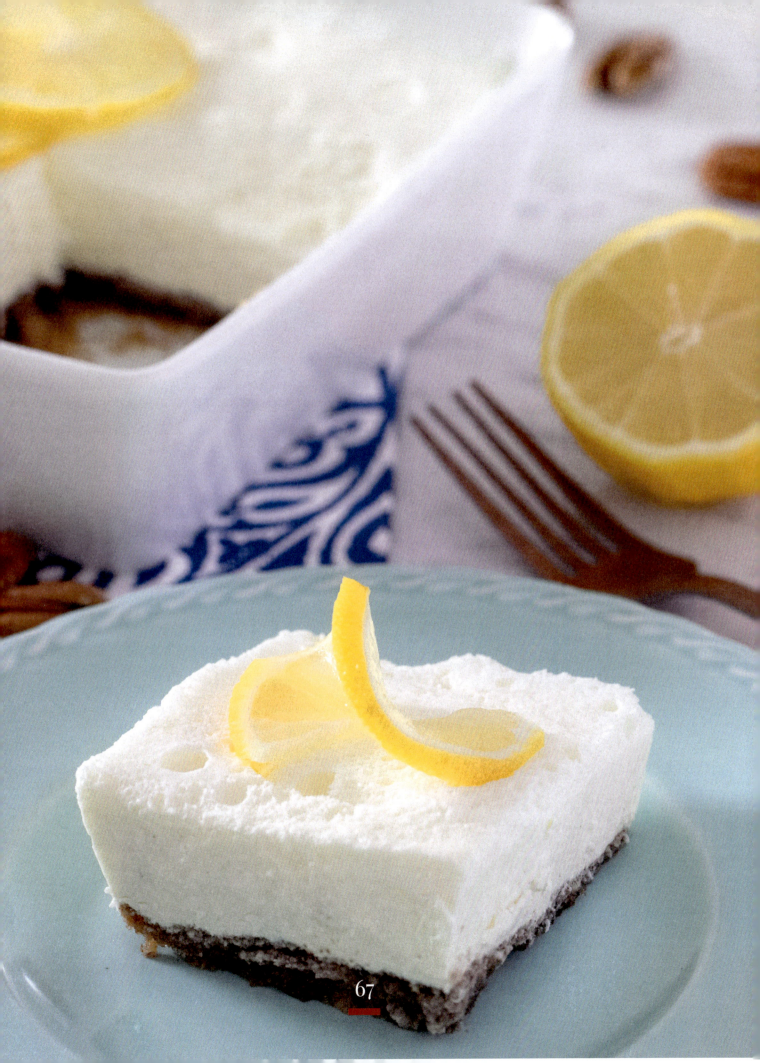

Matcha Soufflé

The robust flavor of matcha pairs perfectly with the light, airy texture of a soufflé. Play around with the sweetness to let more or less matcha shine.

Nutrition

88 calories per soufflé | Makes 2 soufflés

- 8 grams of fat
- 4 grams of protein
- 0.5 grams of net carbs

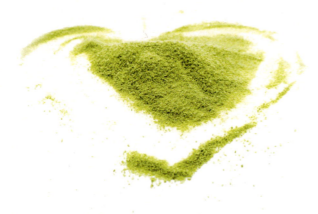

Prep Time: 12 mins | Cook Time: 15 mins

Ingredients

- 1 large egg, separated
- ½ tsp. baking powder
- 1 tbsp. unsalted butter, melted
- 2 tbsp. powdered erythritol
- ¾ tsp. matcha powder

Instructions

1. Beat the egg white with an electric hand mixer until foamy. Add the baking powder and beat until stiff peaks form.
2. Beat the egg yolk with the melted butter, erythritol, matcha powder and a pinch of salt.
3. Very gently, fold in the egg whites into the matcha mixture egg yolk mixture.
4. Liberally grease 2 ramekins with butter and evenly divide in the soufflé batter into each.
5. Bake for 15 minutes at 325°F and serve immediately. They will begin to deflate right away so it's best to finish baking right before eating.

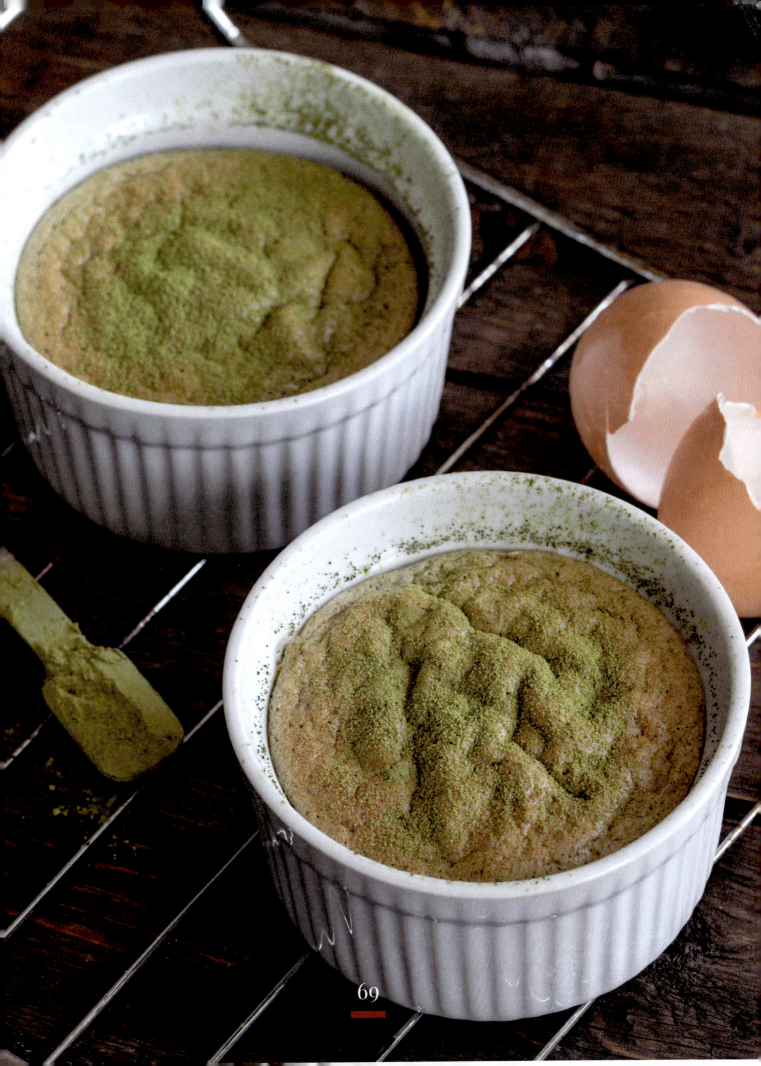

Key Lime Panna Cotta

An impressive dessert made with the simplest ingredients. Think of it as a deconstructed, creamy key lime pie. You'll love the fun texture!

Nutrition

445 calories per serving | Makes 4 servings

- 44 grams of fat
- 3 grams of protein
- 5 grams of net carbs

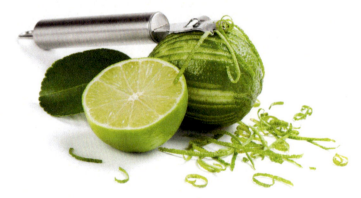

🕑 **Prep Time: 10 mins | Cook Time: 0 mins**

Ingredients

- ¼ cup granular erythritol
- 1 packet (8 grams) unflavored gelatin
- 2 cups heavy cream
- 4 key limes, zested and juiced
- ¼ cup almond meal (or almond flour)

Instructions

1. Add the erythritol and gelatin to the heavy cream in a small pot and heat gently until both are dissolved.
2. Pour in the juice and zest of the key limes (or 2 large regular limes). Add a pinch of salt as well.
3. Grease 4 ramekins (or similar containers of choice) and pour in the panna cotta batter.
4. Chill for 4–6 hours in the refrigerator or overnight.
5. Toast the almond meal in a dry pan on low heat until lightly browned. Sprinkle and serve!

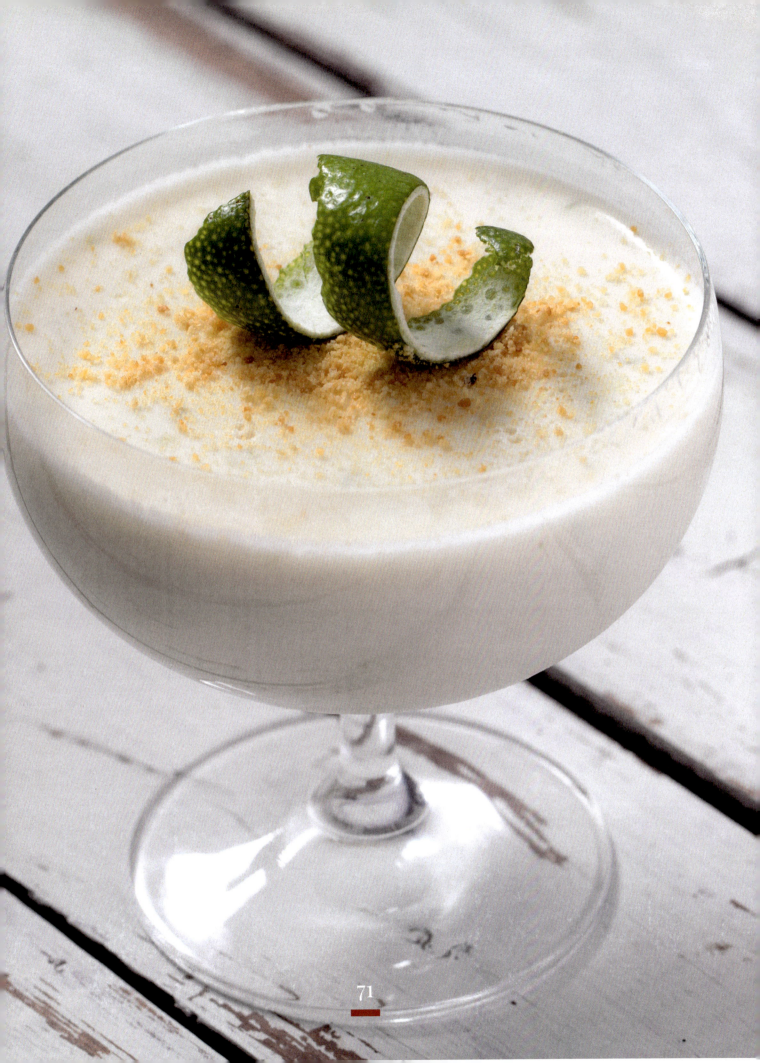

Maple Pecan Cookies

Can you imagine cookies made with only 5 ingredients? We created a deliciously toasty recipe using our trusty, low-carb, high-fat favorite nut!

Nutrition

140 calories per cookie | Makes 12 cookies

- 14 grams of fat
- 2 grams of protein
- 2 grams of net carbs

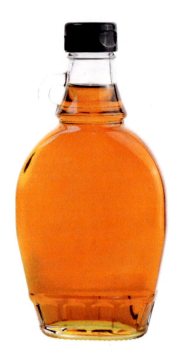

⏱ **Prep Time: 10 mins | Cook Time: 23 mins**

Ingredients

- 2 cups whole pecans
- 2 tbsp. sugar-free maple syrup
- 10 drops liquid stevia
- ½ tsp. ground cinnamon
- 1 large egg

Instructions

1. Toast the pecans on a baking sheet at 350°F for about 8 minutes or until lightly browned.
2. Add the pecans into a food processor and blend until they start to resemble nut butter.
3. Add in the sugar-free maple syrup, liquid stevia, cinnamon, egg and a pinch of salt. Blend again to fully incorporate.
4. Shape the dough into 12 balls, flatten slightly and add a whole pecan onto each. Bake for 15 minutes at 350°F.
5. Let cool completely before enjoying.

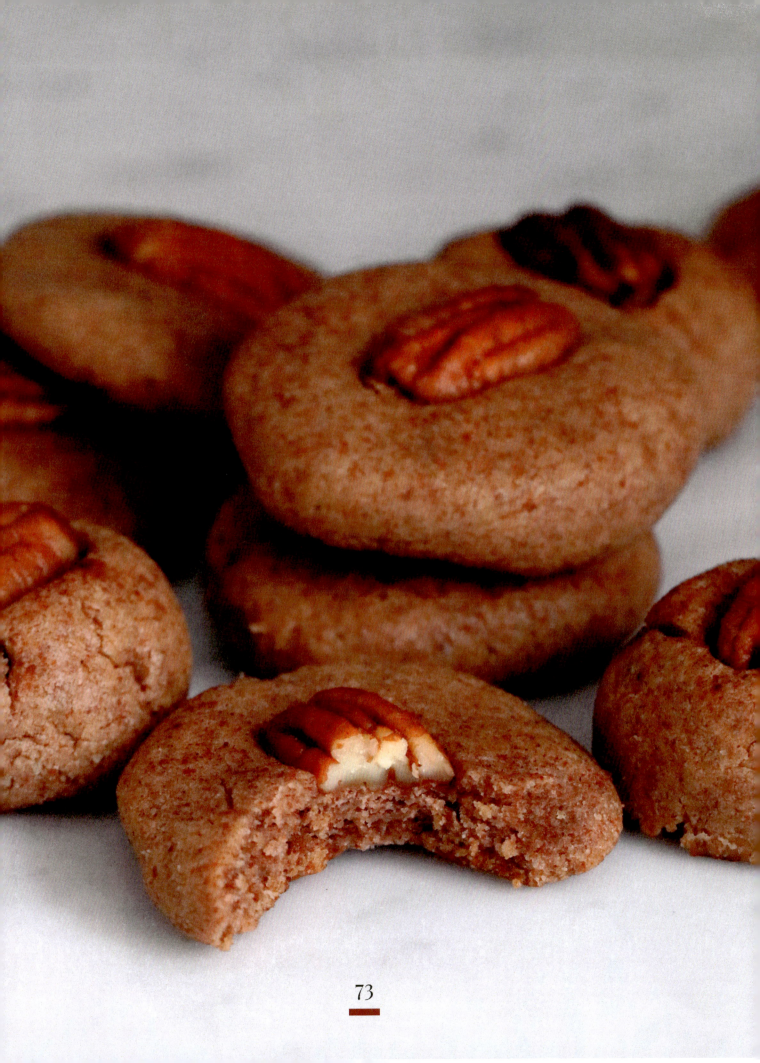

0-Carb Gummy Candy

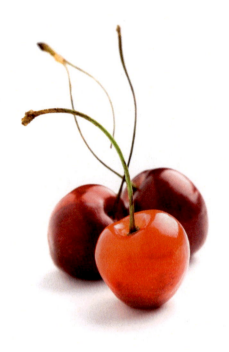

Gelatin is quite versatile. Playing around with the proportion of gelatin and water will give you these fun, sugar-free gummy candies!

Nutrition

9 calories per gummy | Makes 24 gummies

- 0 grams of fat
- 1 gram of protein
- 0 grams of net carbs

🕐 **Prep Time:** 10 mins | **Cook Time:** 0 mins

Ingredients

- 3 packets (24 grams) unflavored gelatin
- ¾ cup cold water
- 1 packet (8.5 grams) sugar-free lemon Jell-O
- 1 packet (8.5 grams) sugar-free cherry Jell-O
- 1 packet (8.5 grams) sugar-free lime Jell-O

Instructions

1. Add 1 packet of gelatin, ¼ cup water and one flavor of Jell-O to a small saucepan over a low heat. Stir until all granules have dissolved, about 2-5 minutes.
2. Spoon or pour the mixture into a silicone candy mold of your choice.
3. Repeat this process for the other 2 flavors.
4. Let the gummy candies cool for a few minutes and then place them in the refrigerator for about 30 minutes to set.
5. Remove them from their molds and enjoy!

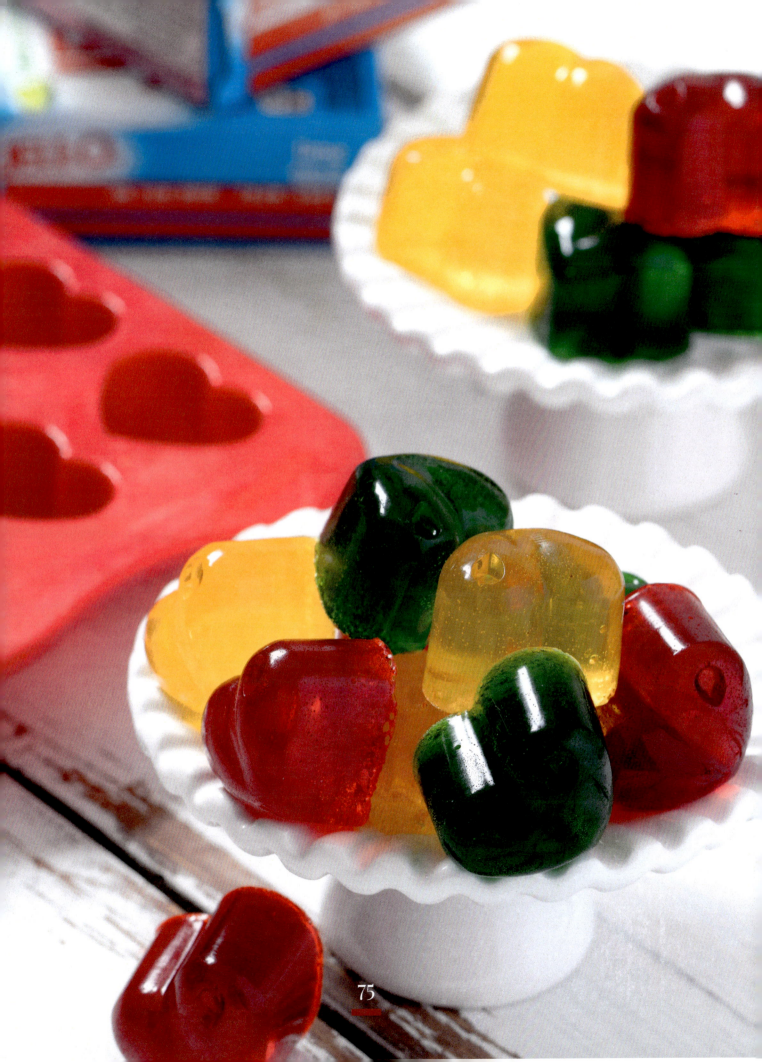

Chocolate Haystack Cookies

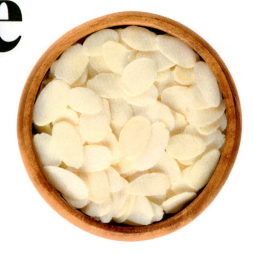

We loved the unique texture of these chocolate haystack cookies and we think you will too! Chewy, chocolatey and delicious!

Nutrition

300 calories per cookie | Makes 6 cookies

- 30 grams of fat
- 3.5 grams of protein
- 5 grams of net carbs

Prep Time: 25 mins | Cook Time: 25 mins

Ingredients

- 1 cup heavy cream
- 3 tbsp. granular erythritol
- 75 grams unsweetened shredded coconut
- 30 grams sliced almonds
- 84 grams sugar-free chocolate chips

Instructions

1. In a sauce pan on a medium heat, combine the heavy cream and erythritol. Once at a boil, lower the heat to a simmer and reduce until it's about half, about 15 minutes.
2. Mix the rest of the ingredients in a bowl. Then, add in the hot condensed cream and stir well.
3. Add the dough to a muffin tin and press each cookie down slightly.
4. Bake for about 25 minutes at 325°F. Let cookies rest for at least 30 minutes before eating.

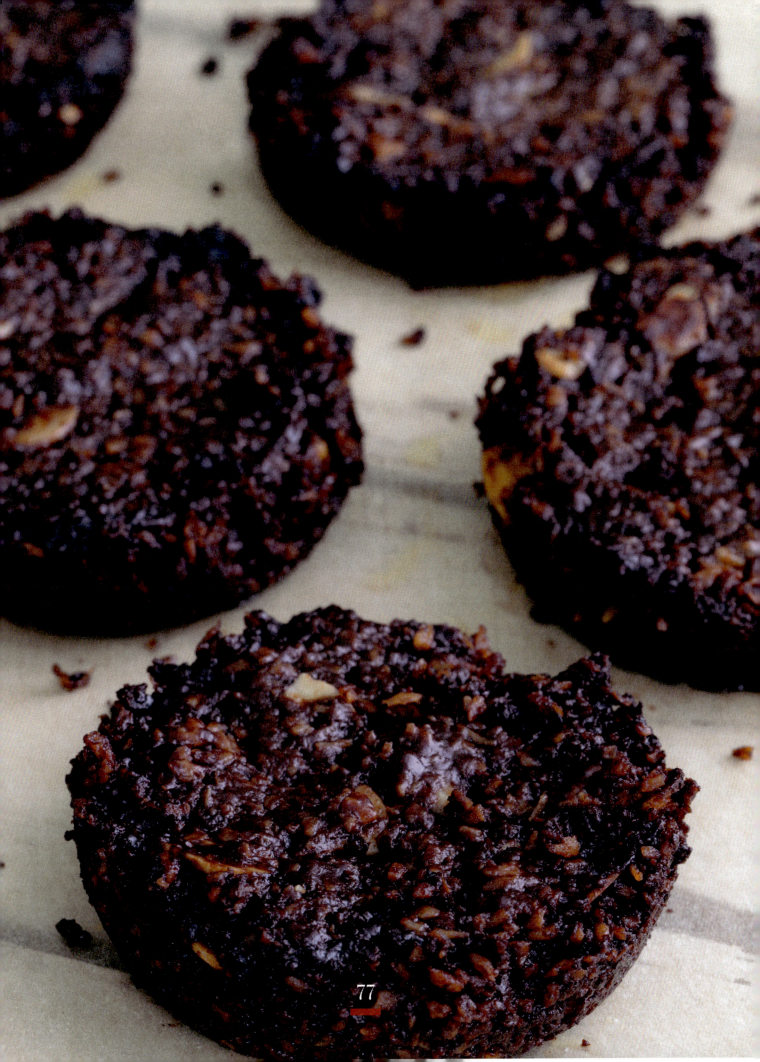

White Chocolate Cashew Clusters

Just 5 easy-to-find ingredients and you'll be enjoying this creamy, crunchy snack with tons of flavor and fat! It's worth the effort to make them.

Nutrition

72 calories per cluster | Makes 12 clusters

- 6.5 grams of fat
- 1 gram of protein
- 1.5 grams of net carbs

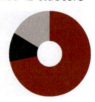

Prep Time: 30 mins | Cook Time: 0 mins

Ingredients

- 36 whole cashews
- 12 sugar-free hard caramel candies
- 50 grams cocoa butter
- 2 tbsp. powdered erythritol
- Pink sea salt to taste

Instructions

1. Toast cashews on a parchment paper-lined baking sheet at 350°F for 5–10 minutes (optional).
2. Arrange the toasted cashews in piles of 3 and add a caramel candy onto each pile. Bake until each caramel is just slightly melted over each nut.
3. Melt the cocoa butter and erythritol and then allow to cool until it's a spoonable consistency.
4. Spoon a bit of the white chocolate mixture onto each cooled cashew cluster and top with some pink salt while still wet. Cool in the refrigerator until hardened and enjoy!

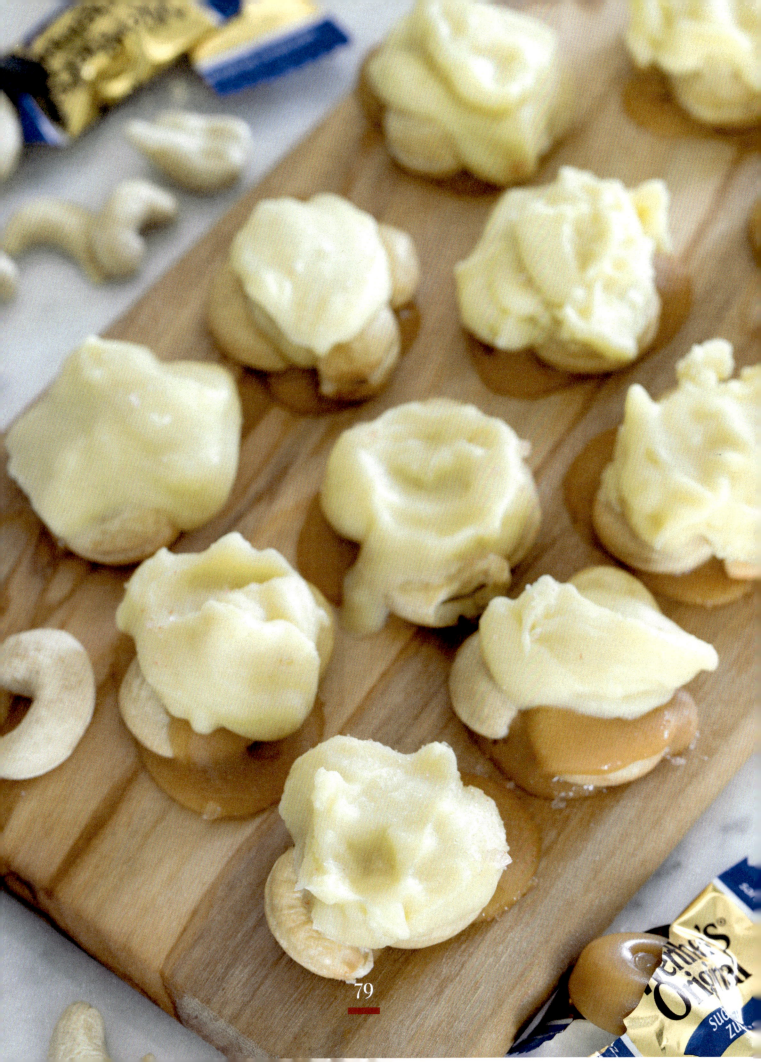

Strawberry Shortcake

A classic strawberry shortcake recipe you can make in no time. We used our trusty Oopsie Roll recipe to make this recipe fun and easy.

Nutrition

308 calories per cake | Makes 2 shortcakes

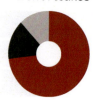

- 30 grams of fat
- 6 grams of protein
- 5 grams of net carbs

🕐 **Prep Time: 20 mins | Cook Time: 25 mins**

Ingredients

- 100 grams strawberries, hulled
- 3 tbsp. powdered erythritol
- 1 large egg, separated
- 1 oz. cream cheese
- ½ cup heavy cream

Instructions

1. Thinly slice the hulled strawberries and mix with 2 tbsp. erythritol in a bowl. Let soak for 30 minutes to release juices.
2. Use a hand mixer to beat the egg white until foamy. Add a pinch of salt, 1 tablespoon of erythritol and mix again until stiff peaks form.
3. Beat the egg yolk and cream cheese until smooth. Then, gently fold the egg white into the egg yolk mixture.
4. On a parchment paper-lined baking sheet, make four 3" circles from the egg batter. Bake for 25 minutes at 300°F. Then, let cool.
5. Beat heavy cream and the rest of the erythritol for about 1 minute. Add the whipped cream to one cake layer, then sliced strawberries and repeat to make each shortcake stack.

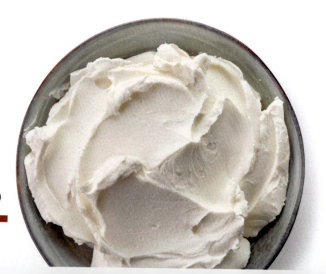

80

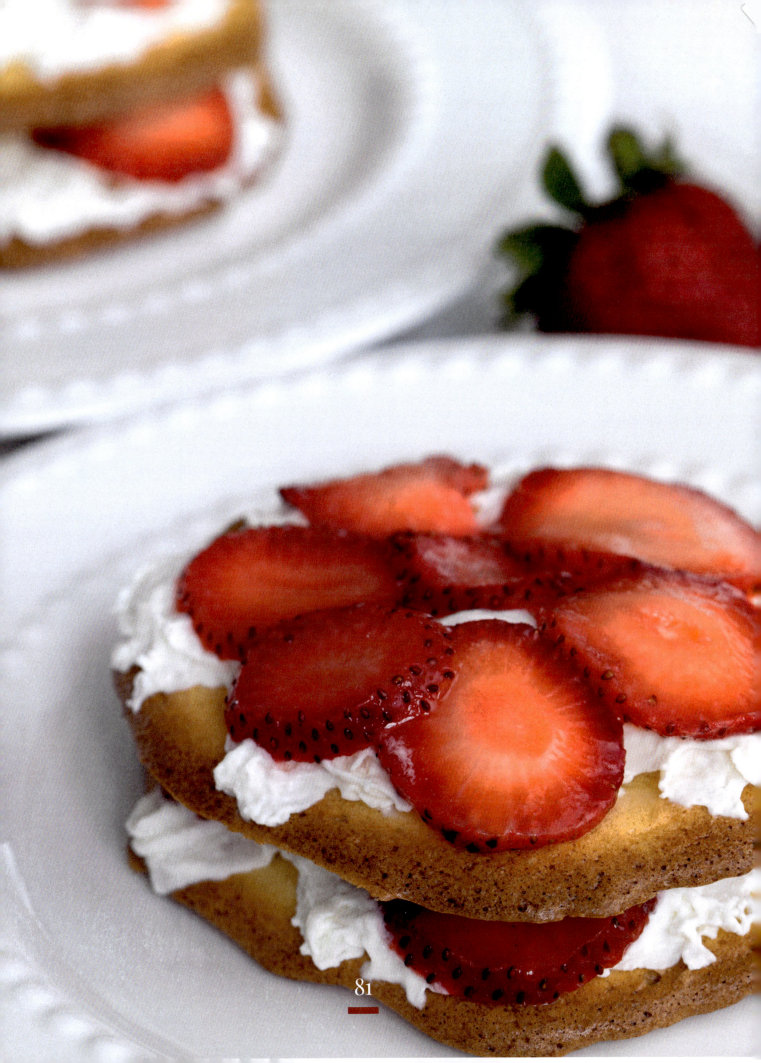

Pumpkin Pudding

It doesn't need to be autumn for you to enjoy some pumpkin every now and then. Keep a can of pumpkin puree in your kitchen for this very recipe!

Nutrition

156 calories per serving | Makes 1 serving

- 14 grams of fat
- 2 grams of protein
- 5 grams of net carbs

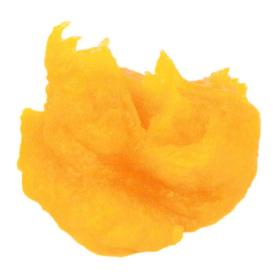

🕒 **Prep Time: 10 mins | Cook Time: 0 mins**

Ingredients

- ½ cup unsweetened coconut cream
- 3 tbsp. canned pumpkin
- 4 tsp. granular erythritol
- ¾ tsp. pumpkin pie spice
- ⅛ tsp. xanthan gum

Instructions

1. Mix the coconut cream, canned pumpkin, erythritol, pumpkin pie spice and a pinch of salt together in a pot on medium heat.
2. While whisking continuously, add the xanthan gum slowly. Heat the pudding on medium heat for 1 minute.
3. Refrigerate for 30 minutes to let it set slightly.
4. Sprinkle pumpkin pie spice on top and serve.

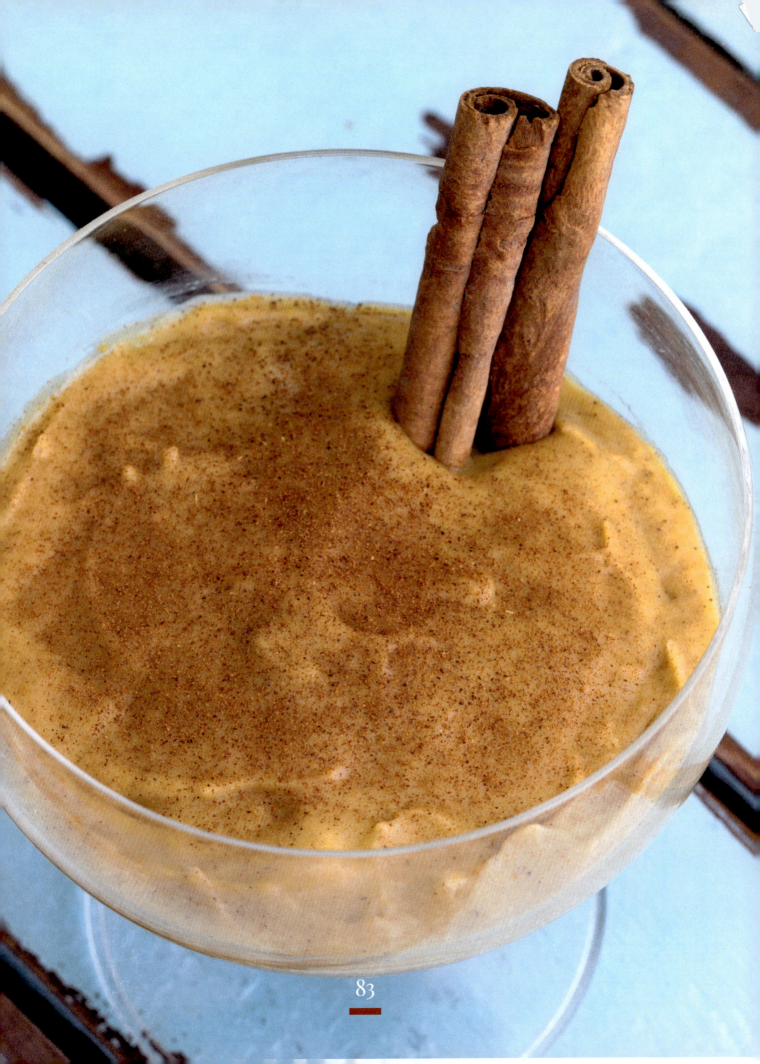

Mint Chocolate Chip Ice Cream

This keto- and paleo-friendly ice cream recipe is dairy-free, sugar-free and artificial coloring-free! The green color comes from the added avocado!

Nutrition per scoop

173 calories per serving | Makes 9 scoops

- 18 grams of fat
- 2 grams of protein
- 3 grams of net carbs

Prep Time: 20 mins | Cook Time: 0 mins

Ingredients

- 20 oz. canned unsweetened coconut milk
- ⅔ cup granular erythritol
- 1 medium avocado
- ½–1 tsp. mint extract
- ½ cup sugar-free chocolate chips

Instructions

1. Freeze your ice cream maker's drum overnight before starting this recipe.
2. In a food processor, blend the coconut milk, erythritol, avocado and ½–1 tsp. of mint extract.
3. Fold in the chocolate chips by hand.
4. Churn the ice cream batter according to manufacturer's instructions. Freeze overnight.
5. Let thaw for 10–15 minutes before enjoying.

Tip: Add 1 tablespoon of vodka in step 2 to keep the ice cream soft after freezing.

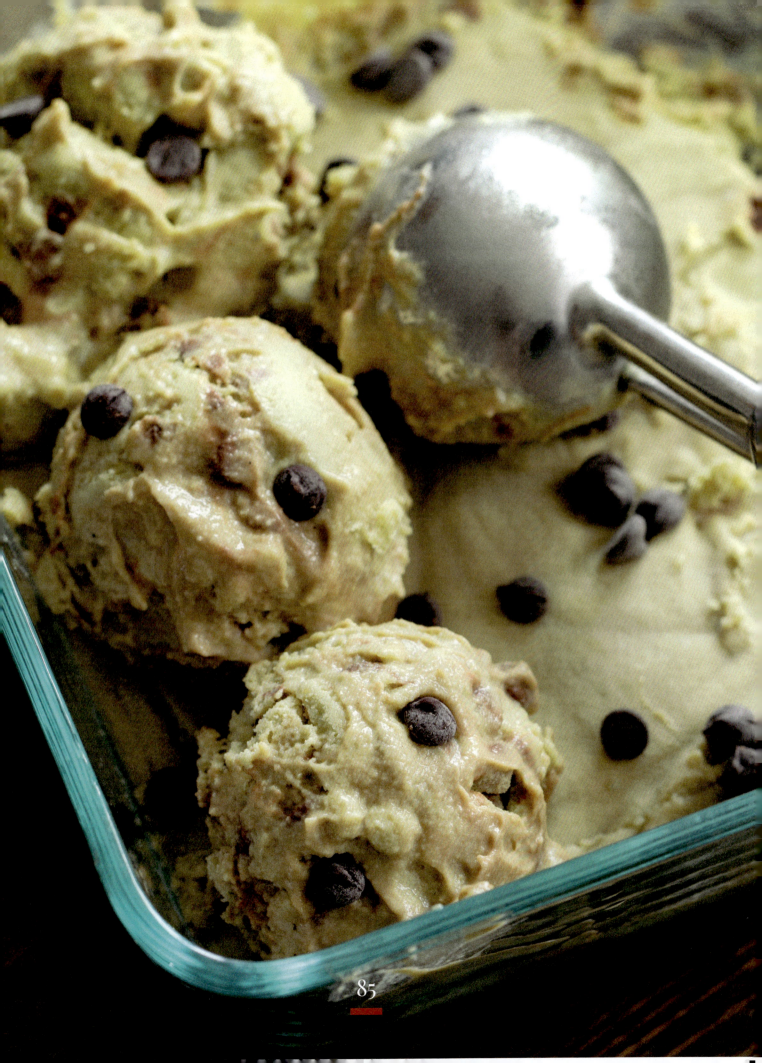

Banana Almond Muffins

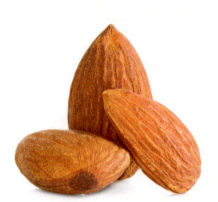

These muffins are sweet enough for dessert but nutritious enough to enjoy as a breakfast too! We toast them up with a cup of coffee or tea!

Nutrition per muffin

289 calories per serving | Makes 6 muffins

- 26 grams of fat
- 14 grams of protein
- 4 grams of net carbs

🕐 **Prep Time: 10 mins | Cook Time: 18 mins**

Ingredients

- 1 cup almond butter
- ⅔ cup powdered erythritol
- 3 large eggs
- ½ tsp. banana extract
- 1 tsp. baking powder

Instructions

1. Use a food processor to blend together the almond butter and erythritol.
2. Then, add in the eggs, banana extract, baking powder and a pinch of salt.
3. Pour the batter into 6 muffin tin cups lined with muffin paper liners.
4. Bake for 16–18 minutes at 325°F. Cool completely to firm up before serving.

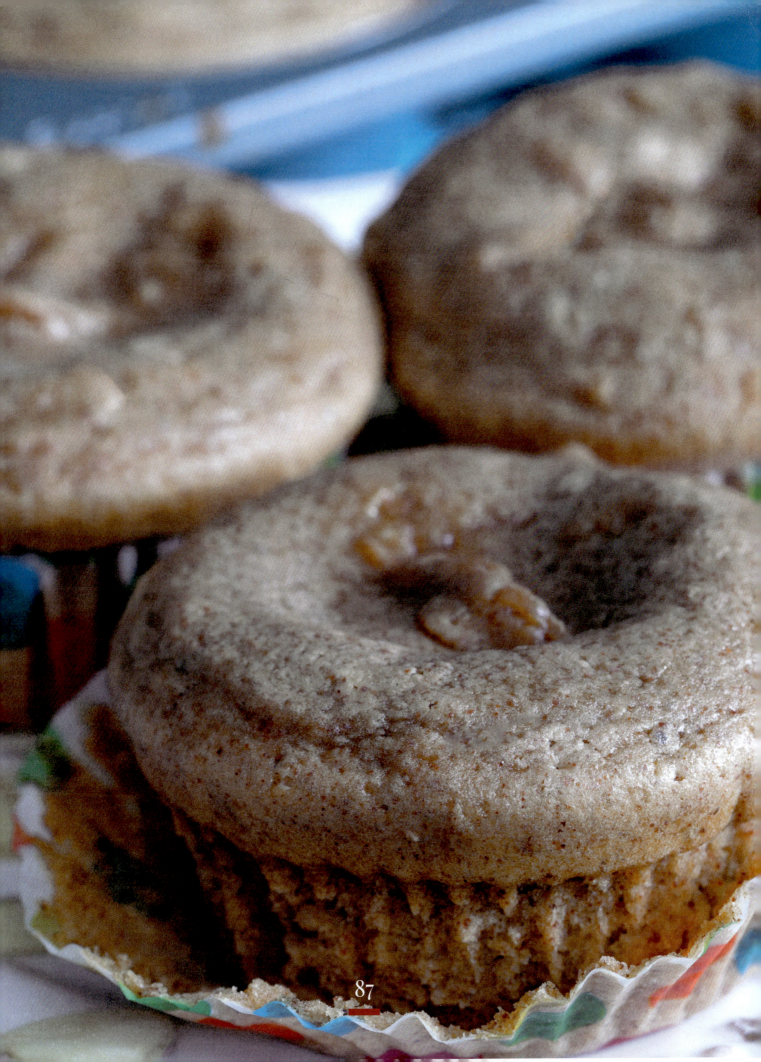

Thank You

Our hopes are that some of these desserts will become staples in your diet making low-carb cooking more delicious and easier for you on a daily basis.

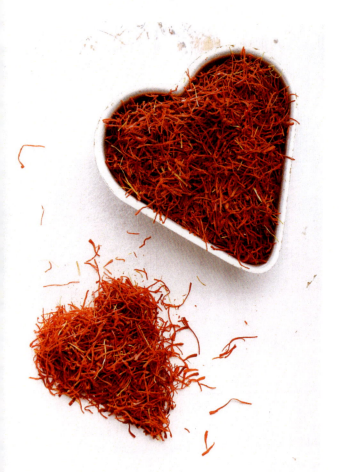

If you have questions, suggestions or any other feedback, please don't hesitate to contact us directly: hello@tasteaholics.com.

We answer emails every day and we'd love to hear from you. Each comment we receive is valuable and helps us in continuing to provide quality content.

Your direct feedback could be used to help others discover the benefits of going low-carb!

If you have a success story, please send it to us! We're always happy to hear about our readers' success.

Thank you again and we hope you have enjoyed *Dessert in Five*!

— *Vicky Ushakova & Rami Abramov*

About the Authors

Vicky Ushakova and Rami Abramov co-founded Tasteaholics.com to provide an easy way to understand why the ketogenic diet is truly effective for weight loss and health management. They create recipes that are low-carb, high-fat and maximize flavor. The books in their *Keto in Five* series are wildly popular among the low-carb community due to their simplicity and efficacy.

Vicky and Rami's mission is to continue to improve their audience's health and outlook on life through diet and nutrition education. They are dedicated to helping change the detrimental nutritional guidelines in the United States and across the globe that have been plaguing millions of people over the last 40 years.

The duo travels the world to explore new cultures, cuisines and culinary techniques which they pass on through new recipes and content available on their website.

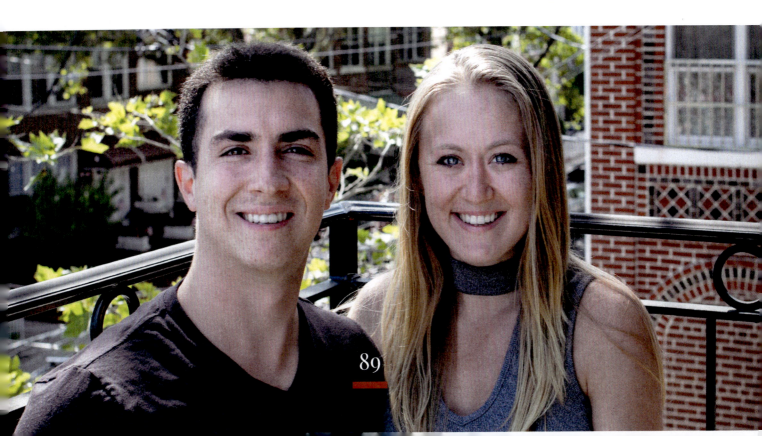

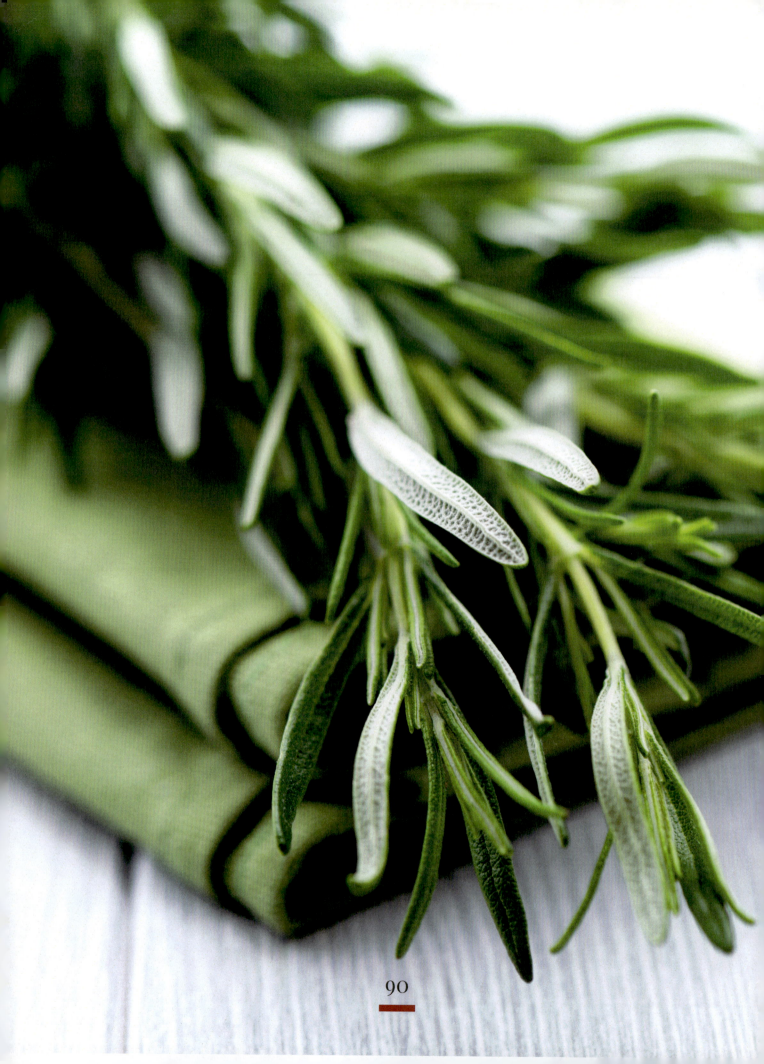

Personal Notes

Use these pages to write down any recipe notes and more delicious ideas.

References

1. Aude, Y., A. S, Agatston, F. Lopez-Jimenez, et al. "The National Cholesterol Education Program Diet vs a Diet Lower in Carbohydrates and Higher in Protein and Monounsaturated Fat: A Randomized Trial." JAMA Internal Medicine 164, no. 19 (2004): 2141–46. doi: 10.1001/archinte.164.19.2141. jamanetwork.com/journals/jamainternalmedicine/article-abstract/217514.

2. De Lau, L. M., M. Bornebroek, J. C. Witteman, A. Hofman, P. J. Koudstaal, and M. M. Breteler. "Dietary Fatty Acids and the Risk of Parkinson Disease: The Rotterdam Study." Neurology 64, no. 12 (June 2005): 2040–5. doi:10.1212/01.WNL.0000166038.67153.9F. www.ncbi.nlm.nih.gov/pubmed/15985568/.

3. Freeman, J. M., E. P. Vining, D. J. Pillas, P. L. Pyzik, J. C. Casey, and L M. Kelly. "The Efficacy of the Ketogenic Diet-1998: A Prospective Evaluation of Intervention in 150 Children." Pediatrics 102, no. 6 (December 1998): 1358–63. www.ncbi.nlm.nih.gov/pubmed/9832569/.

4. Hemingway, C, J. M. Freeman, D. J. Pillas, and P. L. Pyzik. "The Ketogenic Diet: A 3- to 6-Year Follow-up of 150 Children Enrolled Prospectively. Pediatrics 108, no. 4 (October 2001): 898–905. www.ncbi.nlm.nih.gov/pubmed/11581442/.

5. Henderson, S. T. "High Carbohydrate Diets and Alzheimer's Disease." Medical Hypotheses 62, no. 5 (2014): 689–700. doi:10.1016/j.mehy.2003.11.028. www.ncbi.nlm.nih.gov/pubmed/15082091/.

6. Neal, E.G., H. Chaffe, R. H. Schwartz, M. S. Lawson, N. Edwards, G. Fitzsimmons, A. Whitney, and J. H. Cross. "The Ketogenic Diet for the Treatment of Childhood Epilepsy: A Randomised Controlled Trial." Lancet Neurology 7, no. 6 (June 2008): 500–506. doi:10.1016/S1474-4422(08)70092-9. www.ncbi.nlm.nih.gov/pubmed/18456557.

7. Chowdhury, R., S. Warnakula, S. Kunutsor, F. Crowe, H. A. Ward, L. Johnson, et al. "Association of Dietary, Circulating, and Supplement Fatty Acids with Coronary Risk: A Systematic Review and Meta-Analysis." Annals of Internal Medicine 160 (2014): 398–406. doi:10.7326/M13-1788. annals.org/article.aspx?articleid=1846638.

8. Siri-Tarino, P. W., Q. Sun, F. B. Hu, and R. M. Krauss. "Meta-Analysis of Prospective Cohort Studies Evaluating the Association of Saturated Fat with Cardiovascular Disease." American Journal of Clinical Nutrition 91, no. 3 (March 2010): 535–46. doi:10.3945/ajcn.2009.27725. www.ncbi.nlm.nih.gov/pubmed/20071648.

9. "Prediabetes and Insulin Resistance," The National Institute of Diabetes and Digestive and Kidney Diseases. https://www.niddk.nih.gov/health-information/diabetes/types/prediabetes-insulin-resistance.

10. "National Diabetes Statistics Report," Centers for Disease Control and Prevention, 2014. http://www.cdc.gov/diabetes/pubs/statsreport14/national-diabetes-report-web.pdf.

11. Dyson, P. A., Beatty, S. and Matthews, D. R. "A low-carbohydrate diet is more effective in reducing body weight than healthy eating in both diabetic and non-diabetic subjects." Diabetic Medicine. 2007. 24: 1430–1435. http://onlinelibrary.wiley.com/doi/10.1111/j.1464-5491.2007.02290.x/full.

12. Christopher D. Gardner, PhD; Alexandre Kiazand, MD; Sofiya Alhassan, PhD; Soowon Kim, PhD; Randall S. Stafford, MD, PhD; Raymond R. Balise, PhD; Helena C. Kraemer, PhD; Abby C. King, PhD, "Comparison of the Atkins, Zone, Ornish, and LEARN Diets for Change in Weight and Related Risk Factors Among Overweight Premenopausal Women," JAMA. 2007;297(9):969-977. http://jama.jamanetwork.com/article.aspx?articleid=205916.

13. Gary D. Foster, Ph.D., Holly R. Wyatt, M.D., James O. Hill, Ph.D., Brian G. McGuckin, Ed.M., Carrie Brill, B.S., B. Selma Mohammed, M.D., Ph.D., Philippe O. Szapary, M.D., Daniel J. Rader, M.D., Joel S. Edman, D.Sc., and Samuel Klein, M.D., "A Randomized Trial of a Low-Carbohydrate Diet for Obesity – NEJM," N Engl J Med 2003; 348:2082-2090. http://www.nejm.org/doi/full/10.1056/NEJMoa022207.

14. JS Volek, MJ Sharman, AL Gómez, DA Judelson, MR Rubin, G Watson, B Sokmen, R Silvestre, DN French, and WJ Kraemer, "Comparison of Energy-restricted Very Low-carbohydrate and Low-fat Diets on Weight Loss and Body Composition in Overweight Men and Women," Nutr Metab (Lond). 2004; 1: 13. http://www.ncbi.nlm.nih.gov/pmc/articles/PMC538279/.

15. Y. Wady Aude, MD; Arthur S. Agatston, MD; Francisco Lopez-Jimenez, MD, MSc; Eric H. Lieberman, MD; Marie Almon, MS, RD; Melinda Hansen, ARNP; Gerardo Rojas, MD; Gervasio A. Lamas, MD; Charles H. Hennekens, MD, DrPH, "The National Cholesterol Education Program Diet vs a Diet Lower in Carbohydrates and Higher in Protein and Monounsaturated Fat," Arch Intern Med. 2004;164(19):2141-2146. http://archinte.jamanetwork.com/article.aspx?articleid=217514.

16. Bonnie J. Brehm, Randy J. Seeley, Stephen R. Daniels, and David A. D'Alessio, "A Randomized Trial Comparing a Very Low Carbohydrate Diet and a Calorie-Restricted Low Fat Diet on Body Weight and Cardiovascular Risk Factors in Healthy Women," The Journal of Clinical Endocrinology & Metabolism: Vol 88, No 4; January 14, 2009. http://press.endocrine.org/doi/full/10.1210/jc.2002-021480.

17. M. E. Daly, R. Paisey, R. Paisey, B. A. Millward, C. Eccles, K. Williams, S. Hammersley, K. M. MacLeod, T. J. Gale, "Short-term Effects of Severe Dietary Carbohydrate-restriction Advice in Type 2 Diabetes–a Randomized Controlled Trial," Diabetic Medicine, 2006; 23: 15–20. http://onlinelibrary.wiley.com/doi/10.1111/j.1464-5491.2005.01760.x/abstract.

18. Stephen B. Sondike, MD, Nancy Copperman, MS, RD, Marc S. Jacobson, MD, "Effects Of A Low-Carbohydrate Diet On Weight Loss And Cardiovascular Risk Factor In Overweight Adolescents," The Journal of Pediatrics: Vol 142, Issue 3: 253-258; March 2003. http://www.sciencedirect.com/science/article/pii/S0022347602402065.

19. William S. Yancy Jr., MD, MHS; Maren K. Olsen, PhD; John R. Guyton, MD; Ronna P. Bakst, RD; and Eric C. Westman, MD, MHS, "A Low-Carbohydrate, Ketogenic Diet versus a Low-Fat Diet To Treat Obesity and Hyperlipidemia: A Randomized, Controlled Trial," Ann Intern Med. 2004;140(10):769-777. http://annals.org/article.aspx?articleid=717451.

20. Grant D Brinkworth, Manny Noakes, Jonathan D Buckley, Jennifer B Keogh, and Peter M Clifton, "Long-term Effects of a Very-low-carbohydrate Weight Loss Diet Compared with an Isocaloric Low-fat Diet after 12 Mo," Am J Clin Nutr July 2009 vol. 90 no. 1 23-32. http://ajcn.nutrition.org/content/90/1/23.long.

21. H. Guldbrand, B. Dizdar, B. Bunjaku, T. Lindström, M. Bachrach-Lindström, M. Fredrikson, C. J. Östgren, F. H. Nystrom, "In Type 2 Diabetes, Randomisation to Advice to Follow a Low-carbohydrate Diet Transiently Improves Glycaemic Control Compared with Advice to Follow a Low-fat Diet Producing a Similar Weight Loss," Diabetologia (2012) 55: 2118. http://link.springer.com/article/10.1007/s00125-012-2567-4.

22. Sharon M. Nickols-Richardson, PhD, RD, , Mary Dean Coleman, PhD, RD, Joanne J. Volpe, Kathy W. Hosig, PhD, MPH, RD, "Perceived Hunger Is Lower and Weight Loss Is Greater in Overweight Premenopausal Women Consuming a Low-Carbohydrate/High-Protein vs High-Carbohydrate/Low-Fat Diet," The Journal of Pediatrics: Vol 105, Issue 9: 1433–1437; September 2005. http://www.sciencedirect.com/science/article/pii/S000282230501151X.

23. Frederick F. Samaha, M.D., Nayyar Iqbal, M.D., Prakash Seshadri, M.D., Kathryn L. Chicano, C.R.N.P., Denise A. Daily, R.D., Joyce McGrory, C.R.N.P., Terrence Williams, B.S., Monica Williams, B.S., Edward J. Gracely, Ph.D., and Linda Stern, M.D., "A Low-Carbohydrate as Compared with a Low-Fat Diet in Severe Obesity, " N Engl J Med 2003; 348:2074-2081. http://www.nejm.org/doi/full/10.1056/NEJMoa022637.

24. Yancy WS Jr, Westman EC, McDuffie JR, Grambow SC, Jeffreys AS, Bolton J, Chalecki A, Oddone EZ, "A randomized trial of a low-carbohydrate diet vs orlistat plus a low-fat diet for weight loss," Arch Intern Med. 2010 Jan 25;170(2):136-45. http://www.ncbi.nlm.nih.gov/pubmed/20101008?itool=EntrezSystem2.PEntrez.Pubmed.Pubmed_ResultsPanel.Pubmed_RVDocSum&ordinalpos=2.

25. Swasti Tiwari, Shahla Riazi, and Carolyn A. Ecelbarger, "Insulin's Impact on Renal Sodium Transport and Blood Pressure in Health, Obesity, and Diabetes," American Journal of Physiology vol. 293, no. 4 (October 2, 2007): 974–984, http://ajprenal.physiology.org/content/293/4/F974.full.

Made in the USA
San Bernardino, CA
08 August 2018